Antibiotic Interactions

The first of a series of occasional colloquia on aspects of infection which are of current concern to clinicians and scientists.

Medical Society of London
25–28th September, 1978

Antibiotic Interactions

Editor

J. D. WILLIAMS

Professor of Medical Microbiology
The London Hospital Medical College

1979

ACADEMIC PRESS

London New York Toronto Sydney San Francisco

A Subsidiary of Harcourt Brace Jovanovich, Publishers

ACADEMIC PRESS INC. (LONDON) LTD.
24/28 Oval Road,
London NW1

United States Edition published by
ACADEMIC PRESS INC.
111 Fifth Avenue
New York, New York 10003

Second printing 1980

British Library Cataloguing in Publication Data

Antibiotic interactions.

1. Antibiotics—Congresses 2. Drug interactions—Congresses
I. Williams, John David, *b. 1931 (Mar)*
615'.329 RM265.2 79-40948

ISBN 0-12-756350-4

Typeset in Great Britain by Kelmscott Press Ltd, London EC4V 6BJ
Printed in Great Britain by Whitstable Litho Ltd, Whitstable, Kent.

Preface

The publication of these proceedings marks the first of an occasional series of meetings to be held on various aspects of infection. These meetings are being held under the sponsorship of Beecham Research Laboratories and are entitled the Beecham Colloquia.

During the series the committee aim to create the opportunity for multidisciplinary discussions into various key facets of the control of infection.

The first such meeting was held at the Medical Society of London on 25–28th September, 1978, and brought together 25 participants to discuss the development of antibiotic combination therapy and the role of such therapy in the management of infection in man. Ten papers covering selected aspects of combination therapy were presented and much of the subsequent discussions has been included in this book. The papers and discussions not only dealt with the areas of agreement between investigators but also highlighted areas where there were differences in interpretation of data. It is clear also that there are misgivings over some types of combined therapy and it was possible to indicate problems which require further study.

Sir Charles Stuart-Harris
Professor H. P. Lambert
Professor F. W. O'Grady
Professor J. D. Williams
Mr D. Goodchild

EDITOR'S NOTE

Because of problems with the recording of sessions the inclusion of the discussions was only made possible by the skilled interpretation of the tapes by the transcribers and the industry of the participants who clarified their contributions. My thanks are due to all those involved in the above task; and I hope I will not need to apologise for any misinterpretation of the discussions. I also thank Miss B. Tucker who worked willingly and long at the tasks associated with distribution of scripts and collection and inclusion of the corrections.

J. D. Williams

List of Participants

J. F. Acar, Professor of Medical Microbiology, Université Pierre et Marie Curie, Hôpital St. Joseph, 7 Rue P. Larousse, Paris 75014, France.

A. W. Asscher, Professor of Medicine, University of Wales, KRUF Institute of Renal Disease, Royal Infirmary, Cardiff, UK.

Sir Douglas Black, President, Royal College of Physicians, 11 St. Andrew's Place, Regent's Park, London NW1 4LE, UK.

M. R. W. Brown, Professor of Pharmacy, University of Aston in Birmingham, Gosta Green, Birmingham B4 7ET, UK.

W. Brumfitt, Professor of Medical Microbiology, University of London, Consultant Microbiologist, The Royal Free Hospital, London, Department of Medical Microbiology, The Royal Free Hospital, Pond Street, London NW3 2QG, UK.

M. Cole, Head, Biochemical Services Department, Beecham Pharmaceuticals Research Division, Chemotherapeutic Research Centre, Brockham Park, Betchworth, Surrey RH3 7AJ, UK.

W. D. Farrar, Professor of Medicine and Microbiology, Medical School, University of South Carolina, Charleston, South Carolina, USA.

O. J. A. Gilmore, Consultant Surgeon, St. Bartholomew's Hospital, London EC1, UK.

D. Greenwood, Senior Lecturer in Microbiology, University of Nottingham, University Hospital, Queen's Medical Centre, Nottingham NG7 2UH, UK.

G. G. Jackson, Professor of Medicine, Chief, Section of Infectious Diseases, University of Illinois, College of Medicine, P. O. Box 6998, Chicago, Illinois 60680, USA.

E. H. Kass, William Ellery Channing Professor of Medicine, Harvard University, Director of the Channing Laboratory, 180 Longwood Avenue, Boston, Massachusetts, 02115, USA.

J. Kosmidis, Senior Lecturer in Medicine, First Department of Propedeutic

Medicine, Athens University School of Medicine, King Paul's Hospital, Athens 609, Greece.

C. M. Kunin, Professor of Medicine, University of Wisconsin, Veterans Administration Hospital, 2500 Overlook Terrace, Madison, Wisconsin 53705, USA.*

H.P. Lambert, Professor of Microbial Diseases, University of London, Consultant Physician, St. George's Hospital, London SW17 0QT, UK.

E. Larson, Scientific Staff, Division of Communicable Diseases, Clinical Research Centre, Watford Road, Harrow, HA1 3UJ, UK.

J. G. Lewis, Consultant Physician, Edgware General Hospital, Edgware, Middx, UK.

G. E. Mawer, Professor of Clinical Pharmacology, University of Manchester, Department of Pharmacology, Medical School, Oxford Road, Manchester, UK.

F. W. O'Grady, Professor of Microbiology, University of Nottingham, Department of Microbiology, University Hospital, Queen's Medical Centre, Nottingham NG7 2UH, UK.

A. Percival, Professor of Medical Microbiology, Department of Medical Microbiology, The Royal Liverpool Hospital, Liverpool. UK.

G. N. Rolinson, Associate Scientific Director (Microbiology), Beecham Pharmaceuticals Research Division, Chemotherapeutic Research Centre, Brockham Park, Betchworth, Surrey RH3 7AJ, UK.

M. A. Sande, Professor of Medicine, Division of Infectious Diseases, University of Virginia School of Medicine, Charlottesville, Virginia 22908, USA.

J. T. Smith, Professor and Head of Microbiology Section, Department of Pharmaceutics, The School of Pharmacy, University of London, Brunswick Square, London WC1N 1AX, UK.

Sir Charles Stuart-Harris, Emeritus Professor of Medicine, University of Sheffield, Department of Virology, Medical School, Beech Hill Road, Sheffield S10 2RX, UK.

Professor J. D. Williams, Professor of Medical Microbiology, University of London, The London Hospital Medical College, Turner Street, London E1 2AD, UK.

*Present address, Chairman, Department of Medicine, University Hospitals, Ohio State University School of Medicine, 410 West 10th Avenue, Columbus, Ohio 43210, USA.

ORGANIZING COMMITTEE

Chairman—Sir Charles Stuart-Harris, CBE

Professor H. P. Lambert
Professor F. W. O'Grady
Professor J. D. Williams
Mr D. Goodchild

OTHER CONTRIBUTORS TO THIS VOLUME

R. W. Bundtzen, Department of Medicine, University of Wisconsin School of Medicine, Madison, Wisconsin, USA.

F. A. Drasar, Department of Medical Microbiology, University of London, The London Hospital Medical College, Turner Street, London E1 2AD, UK.

P. Gilbert, Department of Pharmacy, University of Manchester, Manchester M13 9PL, UK.

R. Klemperer, Department of Pharmacy, University of Aston in Birmingham, Gosta Green, Birmingham B4 7ET, UK.

Contents

Preface v

List of Participants vii

Antibiotic Interactions 1

SIR CHARLES STUART-HARRIS

Clinical Relevance of Antibiotic Synergy 13

J. D. WILLIAMS and F. A. DRASAR

Pharmacokinetic Interactions of Antimicrobial Agents with Other Drugs 35

R. W. BUNDTZEN and C. M. KUNIN

Laboratory Methods for the Evaluation of Synergy 53

DAVID GREENWOOD

Influence of the Bacterial Cell Envelope on Combined Antibiotic Action 69

MICHAEL R. W. BROWN, PETER GILBERT and RUTH M. M. KLEMPERER

Some Biochemical Mechanisms of Antibiotics Acting Together on Bacterial Folate Metabolism 87

J. T. SMITH

Inhibitors of Antibiotic-Inactivating Enzymes 99

M. COLE

Antibiotic Synergism and Antagonism in Experimental Models of Infection 137

MERLE A. SANDE

The Toxicity of Antibiotic Combinations 151

GEORGE GEE JACKSON

Future Uses of Interactive Chemotherapy 171

H. P. LAMBERT

Index 181

Antibiotic Interactions

Sir CHARLES STUART-HARRIS

Department of Virology,
University of Sheffield, Sheffield, UK.

THE CLINICAL PROBLEMS OF TODAY IN RELATION TO ANTIBIOTIC THERAPY

For some time after the introduction of antibiotics, clinicians were dazzled by their success in the therapy of previously fatal infections. To be able to treat conditions such as staphylococcal septicaemia, which had resisted all previous antibacterial treatment, was a remarkable development. Yet the need to measure susceptibility or resistance to penicillin, shown by its failure against many gram-negative bacilli, encouraged the clinician to consult the laboratory for guidance and to explain his therapeutic results. Consequently when it became apparent that two antibiotics or a chemical with an antibiotic, used together gave better results in the laboratory than one alone, clinicians were quick to change their practice. Two examples from the early phase of therapy with antibiotics will serve as illustration.

Subacute bacterial endocarditis, previously invariably a fatal infection of the heart valves and adjacent endocardium, was included in the early trials of penicillin by the MRC Committee from 1946 onwards (Christie, 1949). Cates and Christie (1951) had collected 442 patients by 1951. Ninety-six per cent of the bacteria recovered from the blood before treatment were streptococci, mostly *Strepto-*

coccus viridans, some enterococci and a few other species. The penicillin-sensitivity of 342 strains was tested *in vitro* for comparison with the concentration of penicillin required to inhibit the Oxford *Staphylococcus*. Most were as sensitive as or more sensitive than the standard to penicillin but a substantial number required up to twice the amount of penicillin and 4% required eight times the concentration. Among the patients yielding the latter organisms there were many who relapsed after treatment even after courses with higher dosage of penicillin. This finding stimulated the acceptance of combined therapy with both penicillin and streptomycin (Cates *et al.*, 1951) originally suggested by Hunter (1947), Robbins and Tompsett (1951) and Jawetz and his group. Indeed Jawetz *et al.* (1950) had shown the synergism of these antibiotics in in-vitro tests on enterococci in the laboratory, and Jawetz and Gunnison (1952) distinguished synergistic from antagonistic antibiotic combinations. This Symposium will pick up this theme without doubt and I shall merely quote from Rahal (1978) who concluded his recent review of antibiotic combinations with the words "Despite a large volume of in-vitro and other experimental data, clinical evidence for synergy or antagonism between antimicrobial agents is sparse".

The second instance of combined therapy comes from the annals of the treatment of pulmonary tuberculosis. The first Report of the MRC Committee concerned with Trials of Streptomycin Therapy in Pulmonary Tuberculosis (1948) contained information concerning the relatively rapid acquisition by tubercle bacilli of resistance to streptomycin. Within a few months of therapy, patients whose initial sputa contained fully sensitive bacilli began to excrete streptomycin-resistant organisms in the sputum. Therapy in these patients also began to fail and it was not until *p*-aminosalicylic acid and isoniazid were added to streptomycin that an entirely satisfactory standard therapy was evolved. Even today when relatively short courses of therapy for 4–9 months based on rifampicin have been found satisfactory, isoniazid, pynazinamide and streptomycin are also necessary (Report of BTTA, 1976; Report of East African and British MRC, 1978). The conquest of pulmonary tuberculosis is, of course, one of the greatest achievements of antibiotic therapy, but the emergence of bacterial resistance during therapy is a key factor in the therapy of many other disorders.

CHANGES IN THE PATTERN OF INFECTIONS

The introduction of antibacterial therapy has been profoundly significant from the standpoint of human ecology. The prophets of doom who spoke of the "honeymoon period" during the 1950s have waited a long time for fulfilment of their forecasts. But the fact that the majority of staphylococcal-infected patients now entering hospital yield organisms which are resistant to penicillin (Hassam *et al.*, 1978) is not without significance for current medicine and surgery. The race for new measures to deal with organisms secreting ß-lactamase has been of critical importance in defeating nature's cunning. Nevertheless the changes observed in the hospital population of severe infections needs to be brought to your attention at an early stage of our discussions.

The Thorndike Memorial Laboratory of the Boston City Hospital has chronicled the changes in the bacterial flora in patients admitted to hospital over many years. Maxwell Finland and his associates have been the driving-force of these reportsand a look atthe findings from 1935 onwards in cases of bacteraemia is instructive. McGowan *et al.* (1975) described the numbers of the annual cases in hospital, the causative bacteria and the case-mortality over the period 1935 to 1972. Table I shows the proportions of the total cases with each of the organisms recovered from the blood, excluding obvious contaminants and anaerobes, and the respective case-fatality rates in four selected years. The gross numbers indicate the continuing importance of bacteraemia due to eachand all of the various species listed and also the surprisingly small proportion of infections whose case-mortality has decreased greatly during the period. Such decreases in the mortality from gram-positive cocci as have occurred are offset by the rising mortality from gram-negative bacilli. Table II shows the percentage distribution of the several bacteria in the same four years and illustrates the same phenomenon. These authors separated community-acquired infections present on admission to hospital from those which developed during illness in hospital from the third day onwards. The latter were relatively common in surgical ward patients whereas

TABLE I.

Bacteraemia.
Occurrence and mortality in selected years from Boston City Hospital.*

Organisms	1935	1953	1963	1972
Str. pneumoniae	100 (78)†	107 (27)	127 (22)	108 (15)
ß. haem. str.	53 (72)	10 (50)	58 (45)	45 (31)
Str. viridans	42 (48)	36 (25)	49 (22)	63 (25)
Enterococci	0	24 (38)	44 (43)	38 (40)
Staph. aureus	66 (47)	181 (29)	179 (46)	87 (36)
E. coli	27 (37)	63 (48)	114 (45)	97 (38)
Klebsiella—Enterobacter	0	45 (54)	71 (59)	91 (42)
Proteus	6 (5)	56 (41)	32 (69)	32 (59)
Pseudomonas aeruginosa	1 (0)	17 (47)	48 (48)	22 (64)
Candida	0	22 (23)	9 (67)	30 (57)

* After McGowan *et al* (1975).
† Figures in parentheses are case-fatality rates (%).

TABLE II.
Percentage distribution of organisms recovered from cases of bacteraemia from Boston City Hospital in selected years from 1935 to 1972.*

Organisms	1935		1953		1963		1972	
Str. pneumoniae	32·5		18·3		14·6		15·3	
ß. haem. str.	17·2		1·7		6·7		6·4	
Str. viridans	13·6	84·7	6·1	61·1	5·6	52·6	8·9	48·3
Enterococci	0		4·1		5·1		5·4	
Staph. aureus	21·4		30·9		20·6		12·3	
E. coli	8·8		10·8		13·1		13·7	
Klebsiella–Enterobacter	0	11·0	7·7	31·0	8·2	30·5	13·3	34·6
Proteus	1·9		9·6		3·7		4·5	
Pseudomonas aeruginosa	0·3		2·9		5·5		3·1	
Candida	0		3·8		1·0		4·2	
Other	4·2		4·3		16·0		12·9	

* After McGowan *et al.* (1975).

medical wards contained a higher proportion of community-based infections. These bacteriological changes and their accompanying changes in case-fatality indicate the continuing importance of bacteraemia accompanying severe infections such as pneumonia, bacterial endocarditis and meningitis (Finland *et al.*, 1959). On the other hand the case-fatality does not simply reflect a failure of antibacterial therapy, for the age of the host is a major factor in response to treatment. The organisms concerned in fatal cases of bacteraemia in England and Wales have been documented by the Public Health Laboratory Service. The agreement with U.S. experience is shown in Table III.

THE INDICATIONS FOR COMBINED THERAPY

There are four logical indications for antibiotic therapy in combinations:

(i) to prevent or delay emergence of resistance to a single antibiotic;
(ii) to obtain synergic interaction against an organism whose initial sensitivity to available antibiotics used separately is too low for success;
(iii) to treat infections due to multiple causes with a varying initial sensitivity;
(iv) to treat infections in immunologically compromised hosts.

In practice there may be more than one indication for combined therapy in a particular patient. The following are instances of clinical conditions in which various types of combined therapy have been used:

TABLE III.

Bacteraemia 1975–77 in England and Wales.*

Community-derived Infection	Cases		Deaths	
	Number	%	Number	Case fatality (%)
H. influenzae	347	2	34	9·8
N. meningitidis	326	2	53	16·3
Str. pneumoniae	1 102	8	293	26·6
Totals	1 775	12	380	21·4
Hospital-derived				
Bacteroides	959	6	197	20·5
E. Coli	3 678	25	687	18·7
Str. faecalis	1 139	8	226	19·8
Gram –ve rods†	2 544	18	456	17·9
Pseudomonas	505	3	184	36·4
Salmonellas	249	2	45	18·1
Staph. aureus	3 169	22	546	17·2
Staph. epidermidis	524	4	46	8·8
Total Bacteraemia	14 542	100	2 767	19·0

* Reports by microbiologists in England and Wales to the Commonwealth Disease Centre, Colindale, London.

† *Klebsiella* 1147 (20% deaths)
Proteus 787 (20·7% deaths)
Coliforms 176 (13·1% deaths)
Enterobacter 183 (24% deaths)
Acinobacter, Alcaligenes, Citrobacter, Flavobacter, Hafnia, Serratia 251

Preventing the Emergence of Antibiotic Resistance During Treatment

Examples exist particularly among infections by gram-negative bacilli. *Pseudomonas* infections of the respiratory or urinary tracts are particularly recalcitrant to antibiotic therapy. Brumfitt and others (1967) found carbenicillin useful for urinary tract infections due to *Pseudomonas* but resistance to this antibiotic develops in some instances. Acar and Brisset (1975) successfully combined gentamicin or tobramicin with carbenicillin in cases of urinary tract infection with *Pseudomonas*. The success follows the fact that resistance to carbenicillin with gentamicin is not manifest even when the organisms obtained after therapy are resistant to carbenicillin alone (Smith *et al.*, 1970). Andriole (1971) also demonstrated the synergy of the two antibiotics in experimental infections by *Pseudomonas* in rats.

Pneumonia with *Pseudonomas* infections is secondary to various conditions such as burns, peritonitis or malignancy. Aspiration infection by *Pseudomonas* in cases of respiratory failure secondary to chronic chest disease being treated with intubation has become a major hazard of intensive therapy units. Waldvogel *et al.* (1975) used carbenicillin and gentamicin in combination. Sometimes *Klebsiella* infection coexists with *Pseudomonas* and then a second course of cephalothin and gentamicin follows initial therapy with carbenicillin and gentamicin. Another example of respiratory *Pseudomonas* infection, often accompanied by *Proteus* sp. infection, is secondary to chronic cystic fibrosis (Neu and Swarz, 1969).

Obtaining Synergic Interaction

The rise in importance of staphylococcal endocarditis is attributable partly to the decline of rheumatic fever, so frequently the primary source of secondary bacterial implantation. But both in Britain (Schnurr *et al.*, 1977) and the U.S.A. (Lerner and Weinstein, 1966; Garvey and Neu, 1978) staphylococcal endocarditis has become implanted on valvular prostheses and has followed self-inoculation in drug addicts. Penicillin plus methicillin is often combined with fusidic acid or vancomycin and a similar complex of therapies may be needed in cases of fulminating staphylococcal-influenza pneumonia.

Treating Infections Due to Multiple Causes

The postoperative complications of abdominal surgery, particularly involving the intestines, illustrate the need for antibiotic combinations. Anaerobic infections were stressed by Keighley and others (1976), and Klastersky *et al.* (1977) similarly found multiple anaerobic species in wound infections of cancer patients. Colonic operations seem particularly prone to secondary infection with anaerobes and clostridia, bacteroides, fusobacteria and peptococci were all incriminated by Anderson *et al.* (1976).

The use of prophylactic therapy with lincomycin and clindamycin just before abdominal surgery carries the risk of pseudomembranous colitis now shown to be due to *Clostridium difficile* which resists these antibiotics (George *et al.*, 1978; Larson *et al.*, 1978b). Larson and others (1978a) have recently found vancomycin to be useful in treating this antibiotic-induced condition. Metronidazole combined with gentamicin does not carry the same risk as lincomycin and clindamycin and has been used by Feathers *et al.* (1977) to give prophylaxis against anaerobic infection in colorectal surgery. Before leaving this group of multiple infections one must mention the serious condition of gram-negative or bacteraemic shock. The organisms found by Ledingham and McArdle (1978) among 113 patients included coliforms, *Proteus* and *Bacteroides* species. Therapy with gentamicin and lincomycin initially, and later use of carbenicillin, was recommended by these authors but it must be admitted that ensuing renal failure or the syndrome of disseminated intravascular coagulation may yet kill.

The Problem of the Immunologically Compromised Patient

The use of steroids and many new anticancer agents which affect the immunological system and produce neutropenia leads to a large number of complicating infections. The range of organisms concerned is wide and includes bacteria, fungi and viruses. Infection is thus a terrible hazard to the therapy of the primary condition. A prospective randomized trial of three different regimes of combinations of antibiotics has recently been carried out by the Antimicrobial Therapy Project Group of the European Organisation for Research on the Treatment of Cancer (1978). The patients had granulocytopenia and fever following therapy for acute and chronic leukemia, lymphoma, metastases from solid tumours and aplastic anaemia. Only 63% of the episodes in 625-patient trials were proved to be associated with infection and 13% had gram-negative bacteria. The regimes were carbenicillin and cephalothin, carbenicillin plus gentamicin, and cephalothin plus gentamicin. Each regime was said to cure about 70% of documented infections. The danger of enhancing renal failure particularly in older patients was a drawback to cephalothin plus gentamicin.

I quote this study because it seems to me to illustrate one of the fallacies of clinical trials—namely that the addition of more and more patients increases the chances of obtaining the statistical truth. I would rather have a carefully documented trial of 60 patients with good laboratory and adequate therapeutic control than one of 600 patients in whom only about half of the cases of infection could be documented.

CONCLUSION

In this paper the scope of anibiotic combinations in the therapy of human disease has been discussed with particular reference to the causative bacteria. Inevitably this is merely an incomplete curtain-raiser to this Symposium. At least the attempt has been educative to me personally and has convinced me of the importance both to medicine and surgery of the topic chosen for this first Beecham Colloquium.

REFERENCES

Acar, J. F. and Brisset, J. M. (1975). Combinations of antibiotics in urinary tract infections. *In* "Clinical Use of Combinations of Antibiotics", 126–134. (Ed. Jean Klastersky), Hodder and Stoughton, London.

Anderson, C. B., Marr, J. J. and Ballinger, W. F. (1976). Anaerobic infections in Surgery: a clinical review. *Surgery* **79,** 313–324.

Andriole, V. T. (1971). Synergy of Carbenicillin and Gentamicin in experimental infection with *Pseudomonas*. *Journal of Infectious Diseases* **124,** Supplt., S46–S55.

Brumfitt, W., Percival, A. and Leigh, A. D. (1967). Clinical and laboratory studies with carbenicillin: a new penicillin active against *Pseudomonas pyocyanea*. *Lancet* **i,** 1289–1293.

Cates, J. E. and Christie, R. V. (1951). Subacute bacterial endocarditis. Review by Penicillin Trials Committee of MRC. *Quarterly Journal of Medicine NS* **20,** 93–130.

Cates, J. E., Christie, R. V. and Garrod, L. P. (1951). Penicillin-resistant subacute bacterial endocarditis treated by a combination of penicillin and streptomycin. *British Medical Journal* **1,** 653–656.

Christie, R. V. (1946). Penicillin in subacute bacterial endocarditis. Report to the M.R.C. *British Medical Journal* **1,** 381–383.

European Organisation for Research in the Treatment of Cancer (International Anti-microbial Therapy project group) (1978). Three antibiotic regimens in the treatment of infection in febrile granulocytopenic patients with cancer. *Journal of Infectious Diseases* **137,** 14–29.

Feathers, R. S., Lewis, A. A. M., Sagor, G. R., Amirak, I. D. and Noone, P. (1977). Prophylactic systemic antibiotics in colorectal surgery. *Lancet* **ii,** 4–8.

Finland, M., Jones, W. F. Jr and Barnes, M. W. (1959). Occurrence of serious bacterial infections since introduction of antibacterial agents. *Journal of the American Medical Association* **170,** 2188–2197.

Garvey, G. J. and Neu, H. C. (1978). Infective endocarditis: an evolving disease. *Medicine* **57,** 105–127.

George, W. L., Sutter, V. L., Goldstein, E. J. C., Ludwig, S. L. and Finegold, S. M. (1978). Aetiology of antimicrobial-agent-associated colitis. *Lancet* **i,** 802–803.

Hassam, Z. A., Shaw, E. J., Shooter, R. A. and Caro D. B. (1978). Changes in antibiotic sensitivity in strains of *Staphylococcus aureus,* 1952–78. *British Medical Journal* **2,** 536–537.

Hunter, T. H. (1947). Use of streptomycin in treatment of bacterial endocarditis. *American Journal of Medicine* **2,** 436–442.

Jawetz, E. and Gunnison, J. B. (1952). An experimental basis of combined antibiotic action. *Journal of the American Medical Association* **150,** 693–695.

Jawetz, E., Gunnison, J. B. and Coleman, V. R. (1950). Combined action of penicillin with streptomycin or chloromycetin on enterococci *in vitro*. *Science (N.Y.)* **111,** 254–256.

Keighley, M. R. P., Crapp, A. R., Burdon, D. W., Cooke, W. T. and Alexander-Williams, J. (1976). Prophylaxis against anaerobic sepsis in bowel surgery. *British Journal of Surgery* **63,** 538–541.

Klastersky, J., Husson, M., Weerts-Ruhl, D. and Daneau, D. (1977). Anaerobic wound infections in cancer patients. *Antimicrobial Agents and Chemotherapy* **12,** 563–570.

Larson, H. E., Levi, A. J. and Borriello, S. P. (1978a). Vancomycin for pseudomembranous colitis. *Lancet* **ii,** 48.

Larson, H. E., Price, A. B., Honour, P. and Borriello, S. P. (1978b). *Clostridium difficile* and the aetiology of pseudomembranous colitis. *Lancet* **i,** 1063–1066.

Ledingham, I. McA. and McArdle, C. S. (1978). Prospective study of the treatment of septic shock. *Lancet* **1,** 1194–1197.

Lerner, P. I. and Weinstein, L. (1966). Infective endocarditis in the antibiotic era. *New England Journal of Medicine* **274,** 323–331.

McGowan, J. E. Jr, Barnes, M. W. and Finland, M. (1975). Bacteraemia at Boston City Hospital: occurrence and mortality during 12 selected years (1935–1972) with special reference to hospital-acquired cases. *Journal of Infectious Diseases* **132,** 316–335.

Neu, H. C. and Swarz, H. (1969). Carbenicillin: clinical and laboratory experience with a parenterally administered penicillin for treatment of *Pseudomonas* infections. *Annals of Internal Medicine* **71,** 903–911.

Rahal, J. J. Jr. (1978). Antibiotic combinations: the clinical relevance of synergy and antagonism. *Medicine* **57,** 179–195.

Report by British Thoracic and Tuberculosis Association (1976). Short-course chemotherapy in pulmonary tuberculosis. *Lancet* **ii,** 1102–1104.

Report of East African and British Medical Research Councils (1978). Controlled clinical trial of five short-course (four-month) chemotherapy regimens in pulmonary tuberculosis. *Lancet* **ii,** 334–338.

Report to Medical Research Council (1948). Streptomycin treatment of pulmonary tuberculosis. *British Medical Journal* **2,** 769–782.

Robbins, W. C. and Tompsett, R. (1951). Treatment of enterococcal endocarditis and bacteraemia. *American Journal of Medicine* **10,** 278–299.

Schnurr, L. P., Ball, A. P., Geddes, A. M., Gray, J. and McGhie, D. (1977). Bacterial endocarditis in England in the 1970s—a review of 70 patients. *Quarterly Journal of Medicine* **46,** 499–512.

Smith, C. B., Wilfert, J. N., Dans, P. E., Kurrus, T. A. and Finland, M. (1970). *In vitro* activity of carbenicillin and results of treatment of infections due to *Pseudomonas* with carbenicillin singly and in combination with gentamicin. *Journal of Infectious Diseases* **122,** *Supplt,* S14–S25.

Waldvogel, F. A., Girard, J-D. and Regamey, C. (1975). Combination of antibiotics in severe pneumonias due to gram-negative bacilli. *In* "Clinical Use of Combinations of Antibiotics". 90–108 (Ed. Jean Klastersky), Hodder and Stoughton, London.

DISCUSSION

O'Grady Are there any other major areas where combined therapy is indicated that Sir Charles has not covered?

Kass There are some problems in the therapy of pyelonephritis in the rat. The only situation in which bacteriological cures have been achieved in rats with *Proteus* pyelonephritis has been when kanamycin and chloramphenicol have been used in large doses. None of the single drugs so far tested has achieved a complete cure, but the various combinations have not yet been explored in sufficient detail.

O'Grady In the management of human problems are we not in danger with animal models of creating more infections than we actually need?

Kass There is no answer to this. We don't do very well in the treatment of pyelonephritis so we might just as well face the possibility that some of the animal models may give us insights that may be useful.

Asscher I would like to add one indication to Sir Charles' list. In my practice, the commonest indication for combined therapy is that of an overwhelming life-threatening infection. In these cases I would start combined therapy on a "blind" basis so as to cover the widest possible spectrum.

Brumfitt I would like to make a brief note about the combination of trimethoprim and sulphamethoxazole. From February 1978 this ceased to be patented and it is surprising to me that trimethoprim has not been made available alone. It might be appropriate to discuss later some possible combinations with trimethoprim. Nevertheless, I think that we have to recognize trimethoprim as a very important drug and to ask the question as to whether any sulphonamide is a valuable addition to it, recognizing a very high rate of resistance to sulphonamide.

Percival A further important area of synergistic justification is where one is combining two agents because each of these is toxic and a combination may reduce the potential toxic effect of the therapy.

Asscher I think we have got to be very careful in our use of the term synergy. The term lacks precision and could be taken to refer to almost all interactions other than those which are downright antagonistic. Another problem is that drug combinations which are synergistic in a test-tube are not necessarily synergistic in a patient. In the case of sulphonamide–trimethoprim combinations, for instance, you can easily show synergism in test-tubes but it is very difficult to show that synergism occurs in the patient or for that matter that a synergistic effect is needed. Thus, in the treatment of urinary tract infection trimethoprim alone gives every bit as good a result as the combination of sulphonamide and trimethoprim. Even though synergy may occur it may not be relevant to the results of treatment. I feel it is most important that we abandon the use of the word synergy. Instead I would advocate that antibiotic interactions can be threefold—namely, the drugs may potentiate each other, antagonize each other or show indifference.

O'Grady To come to the particular conditions that Sir Charles mentioned, will people accept that combination therapy was necessary or advantageous, beginning with subacute bacterial endocarditis?

Kunin It should be said that we went through the era of combination antimicrobial therapy 15–20 years ago. In many respects it was disastrous because a large number of combinations were put on the market based upon theoretical considerations which actually were misinterpretations of the medical need. The subject is now resurrected at this meeting. It is important to remember some of the lessons that we learned in the past. Many drugs in fixed-dose combinations may appear reasonable theoretically but must be subjected to trial for ultimate determination of true clinical efficacy.

Percival I question the use of combinations in subacute bacterial endocarditis in some instances. It is often recommended that benzylpenicillin and streptomycin should be used in every instance of subacute bacterial endocarditis due to streptococci other than *Str. faecalis*. In my view this ought to be modified according to the sensitivity of the organisms, because for the most sensitive strains then the cure rates with benzylpenicillin alone have been comparable to those in which penicillin and streptomycin have been combined. It is only with more resistant strains including *Str. faecalis* that there is a beneficial effect which seems to have been shown in the literature but not by controlled trial. However, this only appears to be synergic in comparison with the very massive doses of benzylpenicillin which would achieve the same effect if used alone. This is perhaps an example of using a combination of antibiotics to get an effect which can be achieved at the lower dosage of both but could also have been achieved at a much higher dose of one.

Sande With regard to the cost-accounting of medical care, one of the possibilities which we might discuss is that one might shorten the duration of therapy of some infections by the use of combinations of antibiotics. Some of the data recently published in the United States from the Mayo Clinic suggest that perhaps we can reduce the duration of therapy for streptococcal endocarditis from four to two weeks with a combination of penicillin and streptomycin.

Sir Charles There is no doubt that fear of toxic reactions to streptomycin has always been a deterrent to clinicians giving other than a fairly short course. With the Mayo Clinic series there is quite a strong case for giving large doses of penicillins, at least initially.

For the clinician the area is full of ethical problems because everybody who is faced with the ividual patient has not only got to take account of the mortality of the disease but also the possibility of cerebral embolism and hemiplegia, and therefore the desire is to get on top of the infection as quickly as possible and the therapy is compromised to this end.

Percival With endocarditis one understandably gets emotional overtones in choice of treatment. Professor Asscher's comment about wanting to use two drugs in an overwhelming infection is essentially emotional. One always finds combinations and big doses used in matters of the heart, or concerning children. For the same reason it is obviously going to be difficult to conduct any good trials because the sort of clinical situation in which a combination might be thought beneficial is in a very severe infection and always surrounded by a highly charged emotional climate.

Asscher The choice is far from emotional. It is determined by getting the widest possible spectrum until I know exactly what I am actually dealing with.

Lambert We now have a better opportunity to test some of these points we are talking about than we had hitherto. In this room the clinically involved people all work at centres in which a very large number of valve replacements of various sorts are done and in which a large number of shunts are implanted. Microbiologists put a lot of effort into the study of antimicrobial sensitivities in combination in these difficult situations. Is any effort made in the States to do some multicentre studies of the type which have been done in relation to neonatal meningitis? Here we have a group of patients, many of whom come to surgery not necessarily for infections but for dynamic reasons as well. We have a chance to tackle some tantalising problems. How do we use these preoperative tests on combined chemotherapy? How do we evaluate them? Such evaluation must take into account not only the supposed antimicrobial interaction but also the pharmacokinetic aspects. For example, in neonatal meningitis we believed the drugs were being delivered to the site of action but often they were not. In cardiac surgery we have a large group of patients who get combination chemotherapy and who need evaluating with careful microbiology on the bits and pieces which are removed.

Brown We have been talking mainly either about the effect of drugs on drugs or on the patient but what we are trying to do with the antibiotics is not to attack the patients indirectly but to kill bacteria. What are the physiological states of the bacteria in the different sites of different infections? The state of bacteria is just as important as the state of the drug. We have a good deal of evidence about how grossly varied the sensitivity of bacteria can be depending upon their physiological conditions. If a bacterium is about to divide into two it may be in an environment where some essential nutrient is lacking in which case it will manufacture a new kind of envelope, one better able to take up the nutrients it lacks, and the whole of the envelope-associated properties of the bacteria are likely then to be different. Secondly, the growth rate is important because cells which are dividing quickly or slowly are different cells, with quite drastic changes in the structure of the envelope and in their properties. Finally, we are not dealing with individual cells but with some kind of ecological niche of microcolonies covered with slime stuck in a corner somewhere.

Jackson What bothers me is that bacteria in an infection are not in unison and the drug effects may be quite different from the trends shown in a single physiologic state.

It seems appropriate in the first session that we discuss definitions. It might be useful if we related our discussions to the formula of rational justification of the potential reasons for usage of antimicrobial combinations that Sir Charles gave in his presentation.

Often, in fact most of the time, the demonstration of synergy has a pharmacologic or drug concentration basis where potentiation cannot be shown if one of the drugs is used at the optimum concentration or dosage schedule. Is that synergy? If so, it is one of the reasons why there are so few clear examples of clinical synergy. Is there another and perhaps true synergistic action of antimicrobial drugs on microorganisms when there is no limitation of available drug concentration? In that case the addition of the second drug produces an antimicrobial effect that cannot be accomplished with the first or second drug alone. If possible, I would like to distinguish these two in our definitions and recommended clinical applications and evaluations.

Kass I'd like to suggest some of the definitions that have at least been fairly widely accepted. The first is that in the strictest sense "synergy" be defined as representing the augmented effect of two drugs acting in the same metabolic pathway much as the sulphonamide–trimethoprim effect. We don't have a good word to separate that form of unquestioned synergy from the kind of synergy that is more common clinically in which the mechanisms of action of two drugs are different but the effect of one drug is potentiated by the action of the other. We should also make clear that each combination may have different properties with different strains of organism.

Clinical Relevance of Antibiotic Synergy

J. D. WILLIAMS and F. A. DRASAR

Department of Medical Microbiology,
The London Hospital Medical College, London, UK.

CLINICAL RELEVANCE OF SYNERGY

The colloquium is concerned with all aspects of interactions between antibiotics in the laboratory and when administered to man. There are at the present time so many different antibiotic agents available for treatment of infection that one might consider that therapy with more than one would be rarely necessary. The reasons for giving combined therapy have been detailed elsewhere (Garrod *et al.*, 1973). Current enthusiasm for antibiotic combinations has been fuelled by many laboratories showing enhanced activity of antibiotics when they are used together rather than separately to produce an inhibitory or bactericidal effect. Other studies have shown that in-vitro antagonism may occur between two agents. In this paper we review some of the laboratory information which is accumulating at a rapid rate and discuss how relevant these data are to the treatment of patients with infection.

RELEVANCE OF THE METHODOLOGY

Many laboratory tests have been devised to show microbiological interactions between pairs of antibiotics. These range from simple disc testing to full chequerboard titrations of the two antibiotics but it is often difficult, however, to relate the results of such tests to clinical practice. What are the appropriate conditions for measuring the biological activity of the compounds *in vitro* and how to relate these to in-vivo situations? Different antibiotics may show greatest activity at differing pH ranges, e.g. penicillins are more active at an acid pH whereas aminoglycosides show greatest activity in the alkaline range. For synergy testing a medium is chosen which has a compromise pH which may not reflect conditions occurring at the site of infection which could be, for example, in the biliary or urinary tracts.

The choice of inoculum can be crucial in the study of inhibitory activities of antibiotics and in particular with the ß-lactam antibiotics. Using a low inoculum, low inhibitory concentrations (MICs) can be often obtained even with organisms which produce ß-lactamases and high MICs when a high inoculum is applied. Arbitrary inocula that give reproducible results are therefore usually chosen, although such a size of inoculum may bear no relevance to the clinical situation where the actual numbers of bacteria in a particular situation in the host are often unknown. The relevance of laboratory tests for ß-lactam antibiotics is often obscure even when tested singly (Williams, 1977).

Many antibiotics become heavily protein bound by human serum. There is some discussion as to whether or not an attempt should be made to mimic this situation *in vitro* by adding varying quantities of serum to the broth or agar used for sensitivity testing.

Perhaps a closer approach to the effectiveness of combined therapy in man can be obtained from animal studies but animal models of infection have also been widely criticized; they are frequently difficult to transpose to a human in-vivo situation; they can be difficult to devise and death may be due to a toxaemia rather than to true processes of infection by multiplying bacteria; the pharmacology and pharmacokinetics of antibiotics may be very different in animals and man. Despite these criticisms the results which have been obtained from some animal studies, particularly endocarditis, seem to correlate with the results found in man but such conclusions are really retrospective and although such models may then be considered for prospective studies the results obtained from animal models are usually viewed with caution.

Of the in-vitro studies the chequerboard titration method is most frequently used to give a quantitative evaluation of microbiological interactions. The results can best be interpreted by working out the fractional inhibitory concentrations (FICs) of the different antibiotic combinations showing inhibition (Elion *et al.*, 1954) and plotting these as an isobologram (Kerry *et al.*, 1975). Synergy is visualized by a concave isobol and a combined FIC of ⩽0·7 at the point of maximum synergy.

The MIC has become a guide to the probable in-vivo response to a single antibiotic and because of this we have tried to distinguish between synergy *per se* and clinically obtainable synergy (Farrell *et al.*, 1977) especially when organisms may be resistant to one or both of the antibiotics under test. For clinically useful synergy to be recorded the effect should be to lower the MIC of at least one of the agents to a concentration which can be readily obtained in the serum when the antibiotic is administered in the doses usually given for the treatment of infected patients (Table I).

TABLE I.

Results of study of the synergistic action of trimethoprim and rifampicin to show the difference between "microbiological synergy" and "clinically useful synergy" (modified from Farrell *et al.*, 1977).

	No. of strains	Range of MIC (μg ml⁻¹) to Trimethoprim	Rifampicin	Total no. of strains* showing synergy	No. of strains showing synergy at Serum† levels	Urine‡ levels
Ps. aeruginosa	6	256–>256	4–32	2	0	2
Citrobacter freundii	7	64–>256	8–32	4	0	4
Proteus spp.	6	1–>256	4–32	2	1	2
Providencia spp.	5	32–256	4–32	3	0	1
E. coli	5	<0·5–256	8–32	1	0	1
Flavobacterium spp.	6	64–128	1	5	1	5
E. cloacae	6	<0·5–64	8–>256	4	0	4
Acinetobacter spp.	6	<0·5–>256	<0·5–64	1	0	1
Alcaligenes spp.	5	8–256	1–256	2	0	2
Serratia spp.	4	<0·5–4	16–>256	1	0	1
Klebsiella spp.	5	<0·5–128	16–32	1	0	1
Total strains	61			26 (43%)	2 (3%)	24(39%)

* FIC = 0·625 or less.
† Trimethoprim 1 μg ml⁻¹ Rifampicin 4 μg ml⁻¹.
‡ Trimethoprim 32 μg ml⁻¹ Rifampicin 16 μg ml⁻¹.

Synergy often is most clearly seen when it is not clinically necessary, i.e. when the organism is already fully sensitive to both the agents being tested. For example, a combination of carbenicillin and gentamicin may be synergistic against gram-negative rods (Anderson *et al.*, 1975) when the strains are sensitive to both antibiotics tested. However, in our study on gram-negative rods resistant to genta-

TABLE II.

Hydrolysis of carbenicillin, azlocillin and mezlocillin by 10 strains of gentamicin-resistant *Ps. aeruginosa*.

Percentage hydrolysis in comparison with penicillin G	Carbenicillin strains showing			Azlocillin strains showing			Mezlocillin strains showing		
	Synergy with gentamicin	No synergy	MIC range (μg ml^{-1})	Synergy with gentamicin	No synergy	MIC range (μg ml^{-1})	Synergy with gentamicin	No synergy	MIC range (μg ml^{-1})
0–20	4	—	32–64	7	—	2–16	5	2	4–32
21–100	3	—	32–>256	3	—	2–16	1	—	8
>100	3	—	16–128	—	—	—	1	—	32

micin and sometimes also to carbenicillin, the frequency of synergy was low. There was no apparent relationship between synergistic activity and the degree of hydrolysis of the penicillin (Table II) (Farrell, *et al.*, 1978).

CLINICAL REQUIREMENTS FOR SYNERGISTIC ACTIVITY

The occasions when synergistic activity would be particularly useful in treating an infection are probably few. Such occasions would be when organisms are sequestered in a relatively protected site or where immune processes are inactive and total eradication by antibiotics is required. Examples of this are infective endocarditis and chronic osteomyelitis. Patients with compromised immunity may also require synergistic combinations when undergoing septicaemic episodes. The requirement of synergistic activity for the treatment of infections such as urinary tract infections or simple pneumonias is hard to justify, the use of multiple antibiotics predisposing the patient to multiple side-effects. It is perhaps a hopeful sign that most laboratory studies with combinations of antibiotics are with agents which could be useful in treating the difficult infections outlined above. However, sometimes one has the feeling that there are potentially useful combinations of antibiotics looking for an indication for their use.

CLINICAL STUDIES ON SYNERGISTIC COMBINATIONS OF ANTIBIOTICS

In contrast to the wealth of laboratory data on synergy, clinical studies in which synergy plays an important role in therapy are sparse. Apart from the special case of tuberculosis most of the available information on the beneficial effects of antibiotic combinations, even when synergy is not the prime consideration, is anecdotal and the information is not gathered as results of clinical trials.

Klastersky *et al.* (1976) report that cancer patients with severe gram-negative infections responded significantly better when synergistic bactericidal combinations of antibiotics were used rather than non-synergistic combinations. Sabath *et al.* (1967) found improved results in patients with bacteriuria when they were treated with combinations of penicillins rather than single β-lactams. McCabe and Jackson (1965) found that a synergistic combination of drugs was significantly better than an antagonistic one in the treatment of pyelonephritis.

Some combinations have found an established place in clinical practice as a result of apparent synergistic activity *in vivo* although true clinical trials have never been carried out. The most notable of these is the use of the combination of a penicillin and an aminoglycoside to treat streptococcal endocarditis. Following the laboratory studies of Jawetz and Gunnison (1950) who showed in-vitro synergistic activity of penicillin and streptomycin against *viridans* streptococci and

Streptococcus faecalis, the combination has had wide clinical use. Similar synergy has also been shown *in vivo* in experimental rabbit endocarditis (Carrizosa and Kaye, 1976; Durack *et al.*, 1974). In man the combination of penicillin and streptomycin has also been used with success to treat enterococcal endocarditis (Mandell *et al.*, 1970). The need to add streptomycin to penicillin in *Str. viridans* endocarditis remains unconfirmed (Watt, 1978) but combined therapy for endocarditis is common. Because of the very high degree of resistance by enterococci to streptomycin, gentamicin is preferred by some cardiologists (Oakley, 1978). Certainly the combination of penicillin and gentamicin gave improved results in animals with endocarditis induced by a highly streptomycin-resistant enterococcus (Carrizosa and Kaye, 1976).

The correlation between experimental endocarditis studies in animals, in-vitro sensitivity testing and treatment of endocarditis in man is striking.

Penicillins and Aminoglycosides

Synergy *in vitro* between carbenicillin and gentamicin or the new aminoglycosides against members of the Enterobacteriaceae and *Pseudomonas aeruginosa* has been recognized for some time (Abdou, 1973; Brumfitt *et al.*, 1967; Klastersky *et al.*, 1972). The combinations have been used to treat septicaemic episodes in neutropenic patients (e.g. Jacoby, 1971; Schimpf *et al.*, 1971). In the Klastersky trial (Klastersky *et al.*, 1976) improved cure rates were obtained when in-vitro synergy was present between the combination of amikacin and carbenicillin which was used to treat some patients. Studies using neutropenic rats infected with *Ps. aeruginosa* showed a similar relationship between in-vitro synergy between gentamicin and carbenicillin and survival rates (Lumish and Norden, 1976). Therefore the synergy of carbenicillin and gentamicin and related compounds appears to have clinical relevance. However, as stated above, if the infective organism is already resistant to the two agents the amount of synergy obtained may be insufficient to bring the susceptibility into the clinically useful range.

Cephalosporins and Aminoglycosides

The amount of synergy seen between these agents is relatively minor and their efficacy in producing a cure will depend little if at all on synergistic effect. The combination of a cephalosporin and aminoglycoside may be given to achieve broad-spectrum antibacterial effect in patients with severe undiagnosed infection. In man this combination may be more nephrotoxic than either antibiotic given alone (Klastersky *et al.*, 1974; Bobrow *et al.*, 1972). In animals this effect is reversed and cephaloridine, cephalothin and cephazolin appear to protect rat kidneys against tubular damage by gentamicin (Dellinger *et al.*, 1976; Luft *et al.*, 1976). The reasons for this protective action in animals but increased toxicity in man have not been explained.

Cefoxitin is a cefamycin antibiotic which shows increased stability to the *ß*-lactamases of gram-negative rods and is active against most gram-negative rods, with the exception of *Ps. aeruginosa* (Birnbaum *et al.*, 1978). Data on nephrotoxicity are scanty as yet. We looked for synergistic activity of cefoxitin with gentamicin against 40 strains of very resistant Enterobacteriaceae, *Flavobacterium* sp., *Acinetobacter* sp. and *Alcaligenes* sp., all resistant to gentamicin. Synergy occurred with only four strains at obtainable serum levels of the two antibiotics (Table III).

TABLE III.

Results of study of the synergistic action of gentamicin and cefoxitin to show the difference between "microbiological synergy" and "clinically useful synergy".

	No. of strains	Range of MIC ($\mu g\ ml^{-1}$) to Gentamicin	Cefoxitin	Total no. of strains* showing synergy	No. of strains showing synergy at serum levels†
Citrobacter freundii	4	256–>256	128–>256	0	0
Proteus spp.	4	8–>256	2–256	0	0
Providencia spp.	4	64–>256	1–4	0	0
E. coli	4	32–>256	2–8	1	1
Flavobacterium spp.	4	256–>256	64	2	0
E. cloacae	5	64–>256	16–>256	2	0
Acinetobacter spp.	4	>256	4–>256	0	0
Alcaligenes spp.	4	32–>256	⩽0·5–256	1	1
Serratia spp.	3	128–>256	32–64	2	0
Klebsiella aerogenes	4	64–>256	2–16	2	2
Total strains	40			10 (25%)	4 (10%)

* FIC = 0·625 or less.
† Gentamicin 4 $\mu g\ ml^{-1}$. Cefoxitin 4 $\mu g\ ml^{-1}$.

Penicillins and *ß*-lactamase Inhibitors

An important mechanism conferring resistance to penicillins is *ß*-lactamase production by gram-positive and gram-negative bacteria. Efforts have been made to block the effect of these enzymes by substrate analogues such as cephalosporin C or methicillin and cloxacillin which act synergistically with degradable penicillins (Crawford and Abraham, 1957; Hamilton-Miller *et al.*, 1964; Sutherland and Batchelor, 1964). Such competitive inhibition although striking *in vitro* is seldom achieved in patients infected with *ß*-lactamase-producing organisms because the concentrations of cloxacillin required are at the several hundred microgram level which is only attainable in the urine. Recently several non-competitive β-lactamase inhibitors have been described, including clavulanic acid (Brown *et al.*, 1976) and CP,45-899 (Pfizer). These substances inhibit at least some β-lactamases, thus rendering them sensitive to a wider range of β-lactam antibiotics. Clinical studies still have to be reported but they appear to offer a new useful synergistic combination of agents.

We have studied the combination of CP,45-899 with various β-lactam antibiotics. Against a series of unusual gram-negative rods mainly resistant to ampicillin there was no synergistic activity and the MIC of CP,45-899 was generally high $\geqslant$256 μg ml^{-1}. The MIC of CP,45-899 for *Bacteroides* spp. was much lower (8–32 μg ml^{-1}) and marked synergy with penicillins was seen against most strains including those producing β-lactamases in large amounts.

Similar synergistic activity was also found against *Haemophilus influenzae* when combined with ampicillin or a range of cephalosporins. This effect was most marked with β-lactamase producing strains of *Haemophilus* and Fig. 1 shows the dramatic reduction in the susceptibility to ampicillin with the very small amounts of CP,45-899.

Fusidic Acid and Penicillins

Fusidic acid is often used in combination and many questions have been raised in regard to the clinical significance of laboratory studies of synergy, antagonism and suppression of resistant mutants.

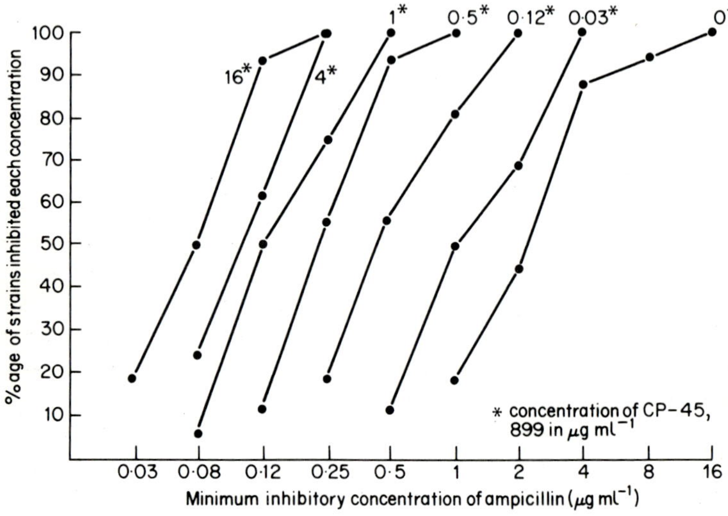

Fig. 1 The effect of varying quantities of CP, 45-899 on the concentrations of ampicillin required to inhibit the growth of β-lactamase-producing *H. influenzae* (A. J. Howard).

Fusidic acid is exclusively directed against *Staphylococcus aureus*. Fusidic acid-resistant mutants are selected with relative ease when this antibiotic is used alone and it is therefore sometimes combined with another antistaphylococcal drug, cloxacillin, erythromycin or lincomycin, to try to prevent this occurrence. Most patients receiving fusidic acid, however, do not receive two antibiotics yet the level of fusidic acid-resistant staphylococci remains low (except when extensive topical therapy has been carried out).

The combination of cloxacillin and fusidic acid has been shown to be efficient in the suppression of fusidic acid-resistant mutants (Barber and Waterworth, 1962) but has frequently been demonstrated *in vitro* to be antagonistic (O'Grady and Greenwood, 1973). *In vivo*, however, the antagonism seems to be insignificant, as good recovery from staphylococcal pneumonias has been reported in patients receiving this combination (Jensen and Lassen, 1969) and, in long-term therapy at least, the value of suppressing resistant mutants outweighs the disadvantages of antagonism.

Fusidic acid is concentrated in bone and widely used in treating staphylococcal osteomyelitis, sometimes in combination with other agents, e.g. erythromycin (McAlister, 1974). Isobolograms made using these isolates showed that in a high fusidic acid/erythromycin ratio the combination was antagonistic. In bone the former ratio would be present and presumably synergy would also be found.

Fusidic acid and rifampicin have also been used in combination to treat staphylococcal infection (Jensen, 1968). This treatment was successful in 33 of 38 patients but rifampicin-resistant staphylococci emerged in two patients.

Trimethoprim and Sulphonamides

Agents which have been extensively studied in combination are sulphamethoxazole and trimethoprim and trimethoprim and rifampicin. Sulphamethoxazole was chosen to partner trimethoprim because the pharmacokinetic behaviour was similar to that of trimethoprim (Busby, 1969). (It does not necessarily follow that sulphamethoxazole is an ideal partner for trimethoprim on microbiological grounds.) The pharmacokinetics of sulphamethoxazole and trimethoprim are the same when given in combination and when given separately (Kaplan *et al.*, 1973). The adsorption of sulphamethoxazole in combination is slightly slower than that when given alone but the extent of absorption is the same. However, when there is a disturbance of renal function the halflife of trimethoprim rises sharply while the rise of sulphonamide is more gradual (Reider *et al.*, 1974).

Although the synergistic activity of trimethoprim and sulphonamides has been unequivocally demonstrated *in vitro* (Supplement, 1973) there is debate on the place of this combination in the treatment of infection. Many of the infecting organisms derived from patients treated with cotrimoxazole are sensitive to trimethoprim alone. Maximum synergy is found only with optimal ratios of the two substances and although such a ratio may occur in urine of patients with uncomplicated urinary tract infection such ratios are not found in bile and are unlikely to be found in tissues due to the differing chemistry of the compounds (trimethoprim being lipophilic and sulphamethoxazole hydrophilic). Sulphamethoxazole may therefore play a redundant role in the treatment of infection whilst giving rise to a significant rate of side effects. Perhaps the use of trimethoprim alone should be considered more widely than at present.

Trimethoprim and Rifampicin

Several groups have studied the microbiological effects of combining rifampicin with trimethoprim because both substances block the biosynthesis of nucleic acids and might be expected to act synergistically. Kerry *et al.* (1975) demonstrated striking synergy with this combination against streptococci and *Proteus* spp. However, although some synergistic effect was found against gram-negative rods, an additive effect predominated. The combination was antagonistic against 24 strains of *Staph. aureus* in the presence of low concentrations of rifampicin.

Grüneberg and Emmerson (1977) demonstrated synergy in only 16 of 100 urinary pathogens and in only 11 instances was synergy present at levels of the antibiotics which could be attained in a clinical situation. Farrell *et al.* (1977) studied synergy of the combination in 61 strains of gentamicin-resistant gram-negative rods and found "useful synergy" in only two strains using attainable serum levels but in 24 strains when attainable urinary levels were considered. These strains included five of six isolates of multiply resistant Flavobacteria resistant to practically all agents available clinically. It appears from these studies that the clinical benefit likely to arise from the synergy is likely to be small except for highly resistant organisms in the urinary tract.

Prevention of resistance is a further justification which has been advanced to support the combination. Kerry *et al.* (1975) found a decreased incidence of rifampicin resistant mutants was in the presence of the subinhibitory levels of trimethoprim; rifampicin resistant organisms were absent from the stools of volunteers receiving a combination of trimethoprim and rifampicin over a seven-day period. Similar results were found by Emmerson *et al.* (1978).

Despite the demonstration of synergistic effect between two antibiotics at a given concentration when two drugs are given together, they may have differing pharmacokinetics. This creates a further deviation from the in-vitro ideal situation.

Several investigations have been carried out in volunteers receiving trimethoprim and rifampicin (Acocella and Scotti, 1976; Emmerson *et al.*, 1978; Hamilton-Miller and Brumfitt, 1976). Using differing dose regimens all found the plasma halflife of rifampicin was significantly reduced when both drugs were given for a week, probably due to changes in biliary excretion. Emmerson *et al.* (1976) also found that the urinary clearance of trimethoprim from serum was significantly increased after eight days whereas clearance of rifampicin was unchanged. These problems may lead to complex dose regimens to ensure that both are present in the serum in appropriate bactericidal concentration at the same time. There is also the possibility that one drug may alter the excretion of the other.

RELEVANCE OF IN-VITRO ANTAGONISM

Most of this paper has dealt with the synergy of two agents and the relevance of reports of antagonism also requires evaluation. Two examples over which some dispute exists are first the antagonism between penicillins and chloramphenicol, and secondly the "dissociated" resistance between lincomycin and erythromycin (Garrod *et al.*, 1973).

REFERENCES

Abdou, M. A. F. (1973). Sensibilität von *Pseudomonas aeruginosa* gegenüber gentamicin, carbenicillin und framycetin. *Arzneimittel-Forschung* **23,** 785.

Acocella, G. and Scotti, R. (1976). Knetic studies on the combination rifampicin–trimethoprim in man. *Journal of Antimicrobial Chemotherapy* **2,** 271.

Anderson, E. L., Gramling, P. K., Vestal, P. R. and Farrar, W. E. (1975). Susceptibility of *Ps. aeruginosa* to tobramycin or gentamicin alone and combined with carbenicillin. *Antimicrobial Agents and Chemotherapy* **8,** 300.

Birnbaum, J., Stapley, G. O., Miller, A. K., Wallick, H., Hendlin, D. and Woodruff, H. B. (1978). Cefoxitin, a semi-synthetic cephamycin: a microbiological overview. *Journal of Antimicrobial Chemotherapy* **4** (Suppl. B), 15.

Bobrow, S. N., Jeffe, E. and Young, R. C. (1972). Anuria and acute tubular necrosis associated with gentamicin and cephalothin. *Journal of the American Medical Association* **222,** 1456.

Brown, A. G., Butterworth, D., Cole, M., Hanscomb, G., Hood, J. D., Reading, C. and Rolinson, G. N. (1976). Naturally occurring *ß*-lactamase inhibitors with antibacterial activity. *Journal of Antibiotics* **29,** 668.

Brumfitt, W., Percival, A. and Leigh, D. A. (1967). Clinical and laboratory studies with carbenicillin. *Lancet* **i,** 1289–1293.

Busby, S. R. M. (1969). Combined antibacterial action *in vitro* of trimethoprim and sulphonamides. The in-vitro nature of synergy. *Postgraduate Medical Journal* **45** *(Supplt)*, 10.

Carrizosa, J. and Kaye, D. (1976). Antibiotic synergism in enterococcal endocarditis. *Journal of Laboratory and Clinical Medicine* **88,** 132.

Crawford, K. and Abraham, E. P. (1957). Synergistic action of cephalosporin C and benzyl penicillin against a penicillinase-producing strain of *Staphylococcus aureus*. *Journal of General Microbiology* **16,** 604.

Dellinger, P., Murphy, T., Pinn, V., Barza, M. and Weinstein, L. (1976). Protective effect of cephalothin against gentamicin-induced nephrotoxicity in rats. *Antimicrobial Agents and Chemotherapy* **9,** 172.

Durack, D. T., Pelletier, L. L. and Petersdorf, R. G. (1974). Chemotherapy of experimental streptoccal endocarditis. II. Synergism between penicillin and streptomycin against penicillin sensitive streptococci. *Journal of Clinical Investigation* **53,** 829.

Elion, G. V., Singer, S. and Hitchings, C. H. (1954). Antagonists of nucleic acid derivatives. III. Synergism in combinations of biochemically related antimetabolites. *Journal of Biological Chemistry* **208,** 477.

Emmerson, A. M., Grüneberg, R. N. and Johnson, E. S. (1978). Pharmacokinetics in man of a combination of rifampicin and trimethoprim. *Journal of Antimicrobial Chemotherapy* **4,** 523–532.

Farrell, W., Wilks, M. and Drasar, F. A. (1977). The action of trimethoprim and rifampicin in combination against gram-negative rods resistant to gentamicin. *Journal of Antimicrobial Chemotherapy* **3,** 459.

Farrell, W., Wilks, M. and Drasar, F. A. (1979). Synergy between aminoglycosides and semi-synthetic penicillins against gentamicin resistant gram-negative rods. *Journal of Antimicrobial Chemotherapy* **5,** 23–30.

Garrod, L. P., Lambert, H. P. and O'Grady, F. (1973). "Antibiotics and Chemotherapy", 4th ed, Churchill-Livingstone, London.

Grüneberg, R. N. and Ammerson, A. M. (1977). The interaction between rifampicin and trimethoprim: an in-vitro study. *Journal of Antimicrobial Chemotherapy* **3,** 453.

Hamilton-Miller, J. M. T. and Brumfitt, W. (1976). Trimethoprim and rifampicin: pharmacokinetic studies in man. *Journal of Antimicrobial Chemotherapy* **2,** 181.

Hamilton-Miller, J. M. T., Smith, J. T. and Knox, R. (1964). Potentiation of penicillin action by inhibition of penicillinase. *Nature (London)* **201,** 867.

Jacoby, G. A. (1971). Carbenicillin and gentamicin. *New England Journal of Medicine* **284,** 1096.

Jawetz, E. and Gunnison, J. B. (1950). The determination of sensitivity to penicillin and streptomycin of enterococci and streptococci of the *viridans* group. *Journal of Laboratory and Clinical Medicine* **35,** 488.

Jensen, K. (1968). Methicillin-resistant staphylococci. *Lancet* **ii,** 1078.

Jensen, K. and Lassen, H. C. A. (1969). Combined treatment with antibacterial chemotherapeutic agents in staphylococcal infections. *Quarterly Journal of Medicine* **38,** 91.

Kaplan, S. A., Weinfield, R. E., Abruzzo, C. W., McFaden, K., Jack, M. L. and Weissman, L. (1973). Pharmacokinetic profile of trimethoprim–sulphamethoxazole in man. *Journal of Infectious Diseases* **128,** 5547.

Kerry, D. W., Hamilton-Miller, J. M. T. and Brumfitt, W. (1975). Trimethoprim and rifampicin. *In vitro* activities separately and in combination. *Journal of Antimicrobial Chemotherapy* **1,** 417.

Klastersky, J., Beumer, J. and Daneau, D. (1972). Susceptibility of *Ps. aeruginosa* to combinations of antibiotics. *Pathologia et Biologia* **20,** 643.

Klastersky, J., Henri, A., Hensgens, C. and Daneau, D. (1974). Gram-negative infections in cancer: study of empiric therapy comparing carbenicillin–cephalothin with and without gentamicin. *Journal of the American Medical Association* **227,** 45.

Klastersky, J., Hensgens, C. and Meunier-Carpentier, F. (1976). Comparative effectiveness of combinations of amikacin with penicillin G and amikacin with carbenicillin in gram-negative septicaemia. *Journal of Infectious Diseases* **134,** S433.

Luft, R. C., Patel, V., Yum, M. N. and Kleit, S. A. (1976). Nephrotoxicity of cephalosporin–gentamicin combinations in rats. *Antimicrobial Agents and Chemotherapy* **9,** 831.

Lumish, R. M. and Norden, C. W. (1976). Therapy of neutropenic rats infected with *Pseudomonas aeruginosa*. *Journal of Infectious Diseases* **133,** 538.

Mandell, G. L., Kaye, D., Levison, M. E. and Hook, E. W. (1970). Enterococcal endocarditis. An analysis of 38 patients observed at the New York Hospital Cornell Medical Center. *Archives of Internal Medicine* **125,** 259.
McAlister, T. A. (1974). Treatment of osteomyelitis. *British Journal of Hospital Medicine* **12,** 535.
McCabe, W. R. and Jackson, G. G. (1965). The treatment of pyelonephritis: bacterial drug and host factors in success or failure among 252 patients. *New England Journal of Medicine* **272,** 1037.
Oakley, C. (1978). Use of antibiotics—endocarditis. *British Medical Journal* **2,** 489.
O'Grady, F. and Greenwood, D. (1973). Interactions between fusidic acid and penicillin. *Journal of Medical Microbiology* **6,** 441.
Reider, J., Schwartz, D. E., Fernex, M., Bergan, T., Brodwall, E. K. Blumberg, A., Cottier, P. and Scheitlin, W. (1974). Pharmacokinetics of the antibacterial combination sulphamethoxazole plus trimethoprim in patients with normal or impaired renal function. *Antibiotics and Chemotherapy* **18,** 148.
Sabath, L. D., Elder, H. A., McCall, C. G. and Finland, M. (1967). Synergistic combinations of penicillins in the treatment of bacteriuria. *New England Journal of Medicine* **277,** 232.
Schimpf, S., Satterlee, W., Young, V. M. and Serpich, A. (1971). Empiric therapy with carbenicillin and gentamicin for febrile patients with cancer and granulocytopenia. *New England Journal of Medicine* **284,** 1061.
Supplement (1973). Trimethoprim–sulphamethoxazole. *Journal of Infectious Diseases* **128.**
Sutherland, R. and Batchelor, F. R. (1964). Synergistic activity of penicillins against penicillinase-producing gram-negative bacilli. *Nature (London)* **201,** 868.
Watt, B. (1978). Streptococcal endocarditis: a penicillin alone or a penicillin with an aminoglycoside. *Journal of Antimicrobial Chemotherapy* **4,** 107.
Williams, J. D. (1977). The correlation of in-vitro susceptibility tests with in-vivo results of antibiotic treatment. *Scandinavian Journal of Infectious Disease* **13** (Suppl.), 64.

DISCUSSION

O'Grady Can I ask whether in "useful" synergy you don't need to test clinically appropriate levels of the two agents. I notice, for example, fixed levels of carbenicillin.

Williams I think 16 $\mu g\ ml^{-1}$ is a fairly useful level for testing carbenicillin. The peak blood level is 60–100 $\mu g\ ml^{-1}$ for a short period of time. We also regard 4 μg of gentamicin per ml as being a "useful" level. It's not feasible to do all those laboratory tests over a very wide range.

O'Grady I'm not suggesting you should do. You think of the level you want to achieve, decide whether it's going to be the peak level or not and test that one.

Percival In considering potential antagonism between chloramphenicol and penicillins, it should be remembered that chloramphenicol is bactericidal against *H. influenzae* and, the chairman has told me, against meningococci. Consequently, for these organisms, antagonism might not be expected. However, as all here know, antagonism between tetracycline and penicillin G was many years ago documented in human pneumococcal meningitis (Lepper and Dowling, 1951; Olsson *et al.*, 1961) and between chloramphenicol and penicillin G in pneumococcal meningitis in dogs (Wallace *et al.*, 1967). These observations are difficult to reconcile with the common, apparently successful, use of chloramphenicol with penicillin and sulphonamide in treating meningitis unless pneumococci behave differently from the other two organisms.

In fact, there are few reported instances of antagonism *in vivo*. I know of a good example in a patient admitted to hospital suffering from acute *Staph. aureus* endocarditis. Addition of chloramphenicol to methicillin was associated with clinical deterioration and positive blood culture (Fig. 1). At this time, the patient's serum inhibited the infecting organism at a dilution of 1 in 64 but was not bactericidal even at 1 in 2. After withdrawal of chloramphenicol, methicillin alone succeeded. The patient's serum was still inhibitory at a dilution of 1 in 64 but was now bactericidal at 1 in 32.

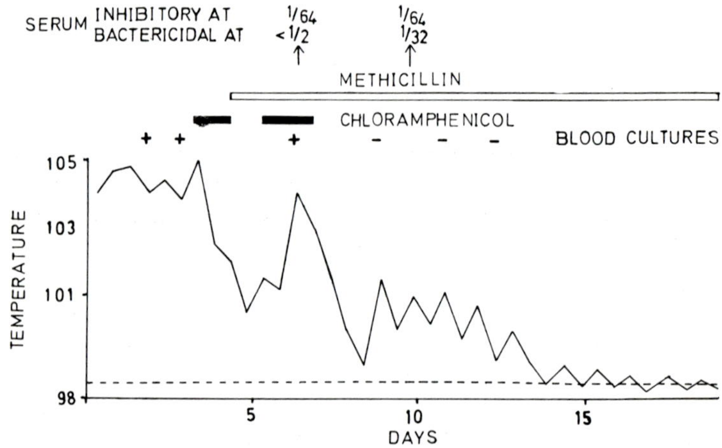

Fig. 1 Antagonism between chloramphenicol and methicillin in a patient with endocarditis caused by *Staphylococcus aureus*.

Brumfitt Trimethoprim went out of patent in February 1978 and already I know four combinations of trimethoprim and sulphonamide.

Studies showed that 1 in 2 combinations, 1 in 5, and 1 in 10 gave the same result, and a ratio of 1 in 20 gives optimal synergy. It rarely does so in the tissues because the volume of distribution of the two is totally different. In acute infections trimethoprim alone has been shown to be as effective as a number of other drugs, including the sulphamethoxazole–trimethoprim combination, with far fewer side-effects. It is also very effective as prophylaxis for urinary infection. I think the time has come for trimethoprim to be available alone, and we know it will be in Europe in the very near future. With sulphonamides the resistance in gram-negative rods in the community is 25% and in hospital practice 50%. Therefore, as Professor Williams has said, in 50% of patients you are in fact using trimethoprim alone.

Why have I chosen to use a combination of rifampicin and trimethoprim? What other drug would one choose to use with trimethoprim which would be as compatible as rifampicin and with no cross-resistance? Synergy is desirable but we don't think it's very important. Rifampicin complements the spectrum of trimethoprim and virtually eliminates all bacteria. It is widely distributed *in vivo* unlike sulphonamides and it is bactericidal. These are some of the reasons we suggested rifampicin and trimethoprim for severe infections of the urinary tract. Rifampicin is rapidly cidal, is active against virtually all pathogens and has a half-life of about $3\frac{1}{2}$ h. In the early stages of illness you need more or less continuous levels of about 50 $\mu g\ ml^{-1}$. If you use a ratio of 300 mg rifampicin + 80 mg trimethoprim there are very few organisms that are resistant. These were the reasons we put forward to the Committee on Safety of Medicines and Drugs, and they were accepted. We are carrying out a multicentre trial in Liverpool, Oxford and in two centres in London. The proof of whether the combination is of value or not will be shown by the results of this trial. It is only being given in difficult cases of urinary or biliary infection.

Incidentally we see no risk of resistance of *Mycobacterium tuberculosis* during a seven-day course of treatment. There is abundant evidence in the literature that this will not occur. Provided a patient doesn't have active tuberculous disease of the chest this is not a danger (Acocella *et al.*, 1977).

Williams The main purpose of my talk is to raise certain areas where synergy is extrapolated from laboratory findings to indicate possible clinical use. Trimethoprim–rifampicin is only one of the combinations which I was calling to question. One of the reasons given for ustwo antibiotics is that it prevents resistance developing to one or other of the drugs; this is correct provided that the antibiotics are both active. When a combination of rifampicin and trimethoprim is used and the organism is already resistant to trimethoprim, resistance to rifampicin emerges in 50% of patients within about four days. This is the type of very difficult patient you suggest treating with combination therapy and I would suspect that quite a lot might have resistance to trimethoprim already.

Sande That is the point that worries me mostly about the combination. Rifampicin probably has a valuable future specifically as an antistaphylococcal drug. A number of papers have recently been published in the United States on its use in patients with infected prostheses. We have used it in four patients who received treatment for a year. We used rifampicin and cloxacillin or other oral agents and compared the serum cidal levels with parenteral treatment with nafcillin or methicillin or vancomycin. The serum cidal levels have been between two and ten times higher on the oral therapy against *Staph. aureus, Staph. epidermidis* and various corynebacteria. I think it has potentially a great future against these organisms. We have also found it useful in the treatment of staphylococcal furunculosis. We again have always used another antistaphylococcal drug. I am worried that using rifampicin and trimethoprim is like using rifampicin alone against staphylococci. Rifampicin-resistant strains may emerge shortening its potential usefulness. So I am concerned about this combination because in the next three or four years rifampicin may emerge as a valuable drug in serious and non-serious staphylococcal infections.

Lambert I was also concerned about this point and would like to ask whether Professor Brumfitt's trials did not include studies of the resistance of the patients' nasopharyngeal staphylococci and meningococci to rifampicin and the other antibiotics.

Brumfitt In our hospital the incidence of resistance overall in gram-negative rods to trimethoprim is only 3%. I have seen the literature on the gram-positives and their resistance is higher in some centres. I agree with you that this is a very serious matter.

Kunin I am disturbed about fixed-dose combinations particularly when resistance may be common in one of the components. One agent might be a superb antistaphylococcal drug. In other instances, it might be an excellent anti-gram-negative. The chances of misuse of the combination are enormous because of the magic of the two names rifampicin and trimethoprim. My hope is that they should not be marketed as a fixed-dose combination but rather used together in certain circumstances where the combination may have special value. For example, there is little need for a fixed-dose combination of rifampicin and isoniazid although they are commonly used in combinat)on.

Brumfitt There are two sides to this story. Patients may be in a confused state when they take the drugs and we have been very concerned that there should be a single fixed ratio. We have decided to try a fixed ratio of 80 mg trimethoprim together with 300 mg rifampicin.

Kunin I would also doubt that the authorities which license drugs would accept fixed combinations of these drugs for a wide variety of infections where a single agent is quite adequate.

Kass It is useful to recall that most combinations that lead to apparent antagonism or apparent synergism produce either of these effects within a fairly narrow range of relative concentrations of the two drugs that are involved. On the other hand, when there is a great excess of either of the two drugs, neither antagonism or synergism can be demonstrated. Clinically, we generally work with substantial excesses above the minimal bactericidal concentrations of either or both drugs. It is not a surprise, therefore, that the clinical demonstration of either antagonism or synergism is uncommon and perhaps unlikely, except in those situations in which limiting concentrations of the two drugs may be involved. Perhaps this is why the only important clinical demonstration of antagonism, demonstrated in the case of penicillin and a tetracycline, was demonstrated for pneumococcal meningitis in which the concentrations of drug in the cerebrospinal fluid tend to be limiting.

One exception to the general statement about the difficulty of achieving limiting concentrations of the two drugs under clinical conditions comes from the studies involving sulphamethoxazole and trimethoprim. In this combination the ratio between the drugs that still permits synergistic effect is wide. Thus, even though the drugs are excreted quite differently and undoubtedly enter and leave body compartments at different rates, the range of ratios that are effective is wide enough to permit one to guess that a synergistic effect will be obtained in most instances in which the combination is used. However, one would feel more comfortable about this combination if the sulphonamide that was linked with trimethoprim had similar properties of absorption, penetration and execretion so that it would be more likely that the two drugs would be present in something approaching the optimal ratio that has been shown to be synergistic.

O'Grady I would like to support that by referring to the study where Greenwood and I looked at the interaction between fusidic acid and penicillin. In that study we examined ten strains: only half showed antagonism; the other half showed various degrees of interaction or indifference. Even among the strains which showed the most marked antagonism, there was still a conventional degree of bactericidal activity in that the count went down to less than 1 in 1000 of the original inoculum. Where laboratory evidence of antagonism was most marked, there was still no reason to believe that that antagonism would be clinically significant. The other point was precisely the one you made about the pharmacokinetics—the distribution of those two agents and their halflives are so different that there can be very little opportunity for antagonism to influence the outcome in the patient even if it were of a significant degree.

Lambert I think that is helpful to our discussions because "synergism" and "antagonism" are often taken to be absolutes and when someone says there is synergy occurring everyone starts using these drugs, and similarly when antagonism is reported people say "we can't use these two agents together any more because there is antagonism". This creates the problem of antagonism between clinician and microbiologist because microbiologists read more into reports of antagonism.

Asscher I would like to underline what Professor Kass said about overtreating infections. To me as a clinician, it always seems preferable to use one drug where one will do. Let us take the example of the combination drug cotrimoxazole. In a recent trial we compared the combination of sulphonamide and trimethoprim with trimethoprim alone and found that using 50 mg twice a day of trimethoprim alone gave the same high cure rate as cotrimoxazole. It follows that the synergy between sulphonamide and trimethoprim is not needed to deal with urinary tract infection in general practice. The use of cotrimoxazole in this situation merely exposes our patients to the additional risk of unwanted effects from the sulphonamide. The only excuse for using cotrimoxazole in the treatment of primary urinary tract infection might be that the sulphonamide component prevents the emergence of trimethoprim-resistant strains but so far as I am aware there is no evidence to suggest that sulphonamides actually do this.

Jackson Professor Williams has addressed the question of clinical relevance and one must observe that in assessing clinical relevance of synergism or antagonism, it is evident that under most conditions the methods for the quantitative measurement of clinical disease and its response to treatment are too subtle and variable for recognition of the effects of drug combinations. Also the doses of one or another of the drugs used are often large, relative to the inhibitory concentration, and can remove the marginal conditions sometimes required for the demonstration of synergy or antagonism *in vitro* and mask its clinical recognition or obliterate the effect itself. Thus, demonstrated clinical relevance is very difficult to obtain.

Nevertheless, certain microbiological drug interactions are regularly reproducible in the laboratory and are therefore valid biological phenomena. If an effect of the combination is expressed clinically, it will be in the direction of synergism or antagonism as demonstrated *in vitro* and thus the laboratory measurements can serve as a proper basis for rational clinical behaviour in antibiotic use in the absence of proof that the clinical effect of the phenomenon will be significant. This can apply to either synergy or antagonism. To show that treatment with a synergistic or antagonistic combination is superior or less than optimal usually requires laboratory tests, such as measurement of a faster or slower rate of bacterial clearance or the post-treatment return of positive cultures. There are several investigations in which such tests have been done to show the clinical relevance of in-vitro synergy or antagonism. However, only in those clinical situations that are demanding enough or sensitive enough or critical enough can one show the clinical relevance of synergism or antagonism by non-laboratory means. The recognition and differentiation of the more obvious laboratory effects which are true and potentially operational biologic phenomena seems to me to be important and relevant regardless of the greater difficulty in showing the usually more obscure and diminished clinical effects.

Kosmidis I would like to contribute to this meeting by giving you a short account of our data on a clinical trial of rifaprim, a combination of rifampicin (R) and trimethoprim (T) at a ratio of 3.75 to 1 versus cotrimoxazole in urinary tract infections. This was carried out in conjunction with Drs G. K. Daikos and H. Giamarellou.

In a randomized controlled study we used three regimens: A, 450 mg R + 120 mg T twice daily, 16 patients; B, 600 mg R + 160 mg T at bedtime, 15 patients; and C, cotrimoxazole, two tablets twice daily, 18 patients. Treatment always lasted 10 days and the usual toxicology studies were performed before and after treatment. Evaluation of result was made three days and four weeks after the end of

TABLE I.
Comparison of the three therapeutic groups.

	A	B	C		A	B	C
Number of patients	16	15	18	Stone/anatomical abnormalities	6 (37·5%)	6 (40%)	4 (22·2%)
Mean age (years)	47·1	43·2	44·3	Functional abnormalities	3 (18·7%)	4 (26·7%)	2 (11·1%)
Males/females	3/13	5/10	3/15	Responsible pathogens			
Mean weight (kg)	67·1	65·1	65·7	*E. coli*	10	6	11
Mean height (cm)	160	166	161	*P. mirabilis*	5	7	6
Diagnoses				*K. pneumoniae*	1	—	—
Cystitis				*Enterobacter* spp.	—	2	—
acute	7	8	5	*Staph. aureus*	—	—	1
recurrent	4	3	7	Pathogens resistant to:			
chronic	1	—	—	S	15 (93·8%)	14 (93·3%)	15 (83·3%)
Pyelonephritis				T	8 (50%)	6 (40%)	4 (22·2%)
acute	—	—	1	R	0	0	1 (5·6%)
recurrent	1	—	—	S + T	8 (50%)	6 (40%)	3 (16·7%)
chronic active	3	3	2	T + R	0	0	1 (5·6%)
chronic active, with recurrent cystitis	—	—	2				
Asymptomatic bacteriuria	—	1	1				

treatment. The three groups were comparable (Table I), although in group C there was a lower percentage of aggravating factors. A prerequisite for inclusion in the study was sensitivity of the pathogen to the combined sulphamethoxazole–trimethoprim disc, as commercially available. Several of the organisms were later found to be resistant to both sulphonamide and trimethoprim, when tested separately, so there was synergy there.

The results are shown in Table II. There were no differences between the two rifaprim groups. At three days results with rifaprim are comparable to those with cotrimoxazole, perhaps better clinically than bacteriologically, but at four weeks we had a higher failure rate with cotrimoxazole expressed both clinically and bacteriologically. Separate analysis of the results in patients with and without aggravating factors showed the same pattern of response to the treatment groups in both categories of patients. In none of 31 patients receiving rifaprim did resistance to R emerge as a result of treatment, even when the organism was originally resistant to T. In three cases of group C, however, resistance to T emerged during treatment, and in a fourth case due to an organism originally resistant to T but sensitive to sulphonamides, resistance to the latter also emerged during treatment.

I remind you though that 90% of the infecting strains were originally resistant to sulphonamides, so actually the third group was treated as though receiving trimethoprim alone.

TABLE II.

Results of treatment of U.T.I. with rifaprim (A and B) and cotrimoxazole (C). See text for treatment schedule of each group.

Treatment Group	Clinical			Bacteriological			
	Cure	Fail.*	NA*	Erad.*	Rel.*	Reinf.*	NA*
Results at 3 days							
A	13	2	1	12	1	3	—
B	13	1	1	12	2	—	1
A + B	26 (89·7%)	3	2	24 (80%)	3	3	1
C	13 (81·2%)	3	2	17 (94·4%)	1	—	—
Results at 4 weeks							
A	13	2	1	9	4	3	—
B	10	4	1	10	4	—	1
A + B	23 (79·3%)	6	2	19 (63·3%)	8	3	1
C	12 (75%)	4	2	9 (52·9%)	5	3	1

*Fail.—failure; NA—not assessable; Erad.—eradicated; Rel.—relapsed; Reinf.—reinfected.

Asscher Is it important that with cotrimoxazole the ratio be only 1 : 1? Why not use sulphadiazine where you will have a synergistic ratio? Here you are using a 1 : 1 ratio and I don't believe there can be any synergy with this ratio.

O'Grady Do you need any synergy? The answer from the clinical point of view seems to be, yes, but I don't know. Careful trials are needed because, as Professor Asscher said, he was really treating a number of his patients with trimethoprim alone because some organisms were resistant to sulphonamide.

Greenwood In considering different formulations of trimethoprim and sulphonamide I do not think that it matters how much sulphonamide is present because when you give normal dosage of trimethoprim there is so much in the urine that the dihydrofolate reductases are completely swamped and the sulphonamides are contributing nothing.

Brumfitt It does matter if there is trimethoprim resistance. The mechanism of trimethoprim resistance is that the enzyme is altered so that it can bypass trimethoprim, so that the MIC goes up. There are trimethoprim analogues available and I understand they will be put on the market.

REFERENCES

Acocella, G., Hamilton-Miller, J. M. T. and Brumfitt, W. (1977). Can rifampicin use be safely extended? Evidence for non-emergence of resistant strains of *M. tuberculosis*. *Lancet* **i,** 740–741.

Lepper, M. M. and Dowling, H. F. (1951). Treatment of pneumococcic meningitis with penicillin compared with penicillin plus aureomycin. (Studies including observations on an apparent antagonism between penicillin and aureomycin.) *Archives of Internal Medicine* **88,** 489–493.

Olsson, R. A., Kirby, J. C. and Romansky, M. J. (1961). Pneumococcal meningitis in the adult. *Annals of Internal Medicine* **55,** 545–549.

Wallace, J. F., Smith, R. H., Gracia, M. and Petersdorf, R. G. (1967). Studies on the pathogenesis of meningitis. VI. Antagonism between penicillin and chloramphenicil in experimental pneumococcal meningitis. *Journal of Laboratory and Clinical Medicine* **70,** 408–418.

Pharmacokinetic Interactions of Antimicrobial Agents with Other Drugs

ROBERT W. BUNDTZEN

Department of Medicine,
University of Wisconsin School of Medicine,
Madison, Wisconsin, USA. .

and

CALVIN M. KUNIN

Department of Medicine,
Ohio State University School of Medicine,
Columbus, Ohio, USA.

INTRODUCTION

Interactions between antimicrobial agents and other drugs are common, but may be difficult to recognize. They often occur in patients who are being treated for multiple problems with a variety of drugs. For example, a woman taking oral contraceptives may become pregnant while receiving rifampicin for treatment of tuberculosis; a slow inactivator of isoniazid may become drowsy while being treated with phenytoin for fits; or a patient being anticoagulated with warfarin may start bleeding when given sulphonamides to treat a urinary tract infection. The likelihood of such interactions is difficult to predict because antimicrobial agents are a diverse group of chemical agents, each of which exhibits its own peculiar pharmacological behaviour. Interactions may occur at one or more of the steps through which a drug is processed by the body. These include absorption, distribution, biotransformation (metabolism), and excretion (see Table I). In addition, antimicrobial agents may interact with each other. This may lead to biologic inactivation and alteration of disposition of the drugs.

TABLE I.

Mechanisms by which one drug may influence the pharmacokinetics of another.

Absorption	Direct binding by formation of salts or chelates Alteration of motility of the gut Alteration of pH of stomach and small bowel Competition for site of absorption
Distribution	Interference with serum protein binding Interference with uptake by major organs Competition for transport by choroid plexus
Metabolism	Competitive binding to ligands Competition for metabolic pathways Enhancement of biotransformation Interference with protein synthesis
Excretion	Competition for active transport by the kidney Alteration of urinary pH and non-ionic diffusion Alteration of rate of urine flow
Direct interaction	Formation of salts in IV fluids or intramuscular sites when mixed Formation of salts *in vivo*

This paper will review the extensive literature on interactions between antimicrobial agents and other drugs. Data will be presented in Tables and will be supported by a comprehensive bibliography.

PHARMACOLOGICAL PROCESSES

Absorption

Absorption of an antimicrobial agent from the gastrointestinal tract depends on the solubility and pK_a of the drug, the intraluminal pH, formation of insoluble

TABLE II.

Drugs that decrease or slow antibiotic absorption.

Antibiotic	Other drug(s)	Mechanism
Tetracyclines	Bi- and trivalent metal cations (including antacids)	Chelation
Tetracyclines	Sodium bicarbonate	Alkaline pH inhibits dissolution
Tetracyclines Pivampicillin	Atropine	Slowed gut peristalsis
Penicillin	Neomycin	Unknown
Griseofulvin	Phenobarbitol	Unknown
Rifampicin	PAS "granules"	Adsorption to bentonite granules

TABLE III.

The effect of antibiotics and other drugs on each other.

Drugs that increase rate of antibiotic absorption.		
Antibiotics	Other drugs	Mechanism
Tetracycline Pivampicillin	Metoclopromide	Increased gut peristalsis
Penicillin G	Cimetidine	Transient achlorhydria (in some persons)
Antibiotics that decrease the absorption of other drugs		
Antibiotics	Other drugs	Mechanism
Neomycin	Digoxin, warfarin	Unknown
Griseofulvin	Warfarin	Unknown

complexes, gut motility, and active transport of the drug (Tables II, III). The best known antibiotic–drug interaction is between tetracyclines and di- and trivalent cations (Neuvonen, 1976). Large doses of tetracyclines also reduce the absorption of iron (Greenberger *et al.*, 1967), both by binding iron and inhibiting protein synthesis by the gut. Sodium bicarbonate reduces absorption of tetracycline (Barr *et al.*, 1971) by decreasing dissolution of the antibiotic in the stomach.

Penicillin G is readily inactivated by acid solutions. Therefore, conditions which raise gastric pH, such as administration of antacids and cimetidine, sub-total gastrectomy, or pernicious anaemia, might enhance absorption of this antibiotic

(Fairfax *et al.*, 1978). Pivampicillin and tetracycline absorption are slowed by atropine and enhanced by metoclopramide, two drugs which affect gut motility (Gothoni *et al.*, 1972). Bentonite, when present as an excipient in PAS granules, adsorbs rifampicin and thereby decreases its absorption in the gut (Boman *et al.*, 1975). Neomycin affects the intestinal absorption of several agents, including cholesterol, digoxin, warfarin, and penicillin G (Cheng and White, 1962; Lindenbaum *et al.*, 1976).

Distribution

Distribution of drugs in the body depends on their ability to diffuse into the intracellular space from the intravascular compartment and to enter cells. Diffusion is governed by binding to serum proteins (principally albumin), lipid solubility, and cellular transport mechanisms (Craig and Kunin, 1976). Displacement of antimicrobial agents from serum protein binding sites tends to increase antibiotic distribution in the body, lower the concentrations in the blood, increase cellular uptake, and increase glomerular filtration (Anton, 1968). In general, these effects are observed principally with highly serum protein-bound drugs, since small changes in the proportions bound markedly increase the amount of free drug. Penicillin and sulphonamides are among the most pronounced examples (Table IV).

Highly bound sulphonamides are well known for displacing binding of toxic agents such as methotrexate, warfarin, tolbutamide, and pentobarbital to albumin (Christensen *et al.*, 1963; Koch-Weser and Sellers, 1976). This may result in serious side-effects such as bone marrow suppression, bleeding, hypoglycaemia, and somnolence (Table V).

TABLE IV.

Drugs that displace highly bound penicillins and sulfonamides from serum albumin.

Penicillins	Sulphonamides
Sulphonamides*	Phenylbutazone
Phenylbutazone	Oxyphenbutazone
Oxyphenbutazone	Sulphinpyrazone
Sodium salicylate	Warfarin
Penicillin "R" groups	Salicylic acids
Novobiocin	Probenecid
Free fatty acids	Tolbutamide

* Highly bound.

TABLE V.

Antimicrobial agents that displace other drugs from serum albumin.

Antimicrobial agent	Other drug	Clinical result
Sulphonamides	Methotrexate	Anaemia, leukopenia
Sulphonamides	Warfarin	Bleeding
Sulphonamides	Tolbutamide	Hypoglycaemia
Sulphonamides	Pentobarbitol	Increased CNS depression
Nalidixic acid	Warfarin	Bleeding
Doxycycline	Pentobarbitol	Increased CNS depression

Although probenecid is believed to increase serum levels of the penicillins by blocking renal tubular secretion, Gibaldi and Schwartz (1968) found that it decreases the apparent volume of distribution as well. They offered several suggestions regarding this phenomenon, but further studies will be needed to provide a satisfactory explanation.

Biotransformation

Most biotransformations occur mainly in the liver and, to some extent, in the kidney and other organs. Some drugs are also excreted into the bile and then into the gastrointestinal tract where they are altered by bacteria in the gut. The metabolites are then reabsorbed.

The principal reactions of biotransformation are classified as synthetic and nonsynthetic. Synthetic or conjugation reactions are the coupling of the drug or its metabolite with moieties such as glucuronic acid, sulphate, acetate, or glycine. Non-synthetic reactions include oxidation, reduction, and hydrolyses. The enzyme systems involved in biotransformation of many drugs are located in the hepatic endoplastic reticulum (liver microsomal fraction). Enzyme synthesis may be induced or enhanced by exposure to substrates. Thus, one drug may stimulate the biotransformation of an unrelated compound which is metabolized by the same enzyme. In general, biotransformational reactions tend to alter lipid-soluble compounds into more water-soluble derivatives. This in turn reduces the distribution of the drug to extracellular fluid and increases its renal excretion.

Rifampicin is of particular interest because it stimulates both its own metabolism and that of many other drugs, although the exact mechanism is unknown (Tables VI, VII). It has been reported to enhance microsomal drug-metabolizing enzyme activity (including drug hydroxylation), alter hepatic uptake and clearance of bilirubin and sulphobromophthalein, and to cause proliferation of smooth endoplastic reticulum of hepatocytes (Kreek *et al.*, 1976). Its use with cortisol, warfarin, methadone and oestrogens must be closely monitored since it tends to reduce the biological activity of these agents.

In contrast to rifampicin, chloramphenicol tends to inhibit drug metabolism, presumably because it blocks protein synthesis of new metabolizing enzymes. It

TABLE VI.
Drug effects on antibiotic metabolism.

Antibiotic	Other drugs	Effects	Mechanisms
Doxycycline	Phenytoin Carbamazepine Phenobarbitone	Halflife decreased	Hepatic enzyme induction
Isoniazid	Pyrazinamide	Isoniazid levels decreased in slow acetylators	Unknown
Rifampicin	Probenecid	Halflife increased	Competition for receptor at liver cell membrane

TABLE VII.
Antibiotic effects on drug metabolism.

Antibiotic	Other drug	Clinical result	Mechanism
Rifampicin	Cortisol	Addison's disease	Hepatic enzyme induction
	Warfarin	Inadequate anti-coagulation	Increased metabolism
	Methadone	Methadone withdrawal	
	Oral contraceptives	Menstrual disorders, pregnancy	
	Bromsulphalein	Slowed excretion	Competition for receptor on liver cell
Isoniazid	Phenytoin	Phenytoin toxicity in "slow" acetylators	Slowed metabolism by liver
Erythromycin	Theophylline	Increased theophylline serum levels	Unknown
Chloramphenicol	Warfarin Tolbutamide Phenytoin Dicoumarol Cyclophosphamide	Bleeding Hypoglycaemia Toxicity Bleeding Incomplete activation	Hepatic drug metabolism inhibited

also increases the blood halflife of tolbutamide, phenytoin, and dicumarol (Christensen and Skovsted, 1969; Rose *et al.*, 1977). Chloramphenicol interferes with the action of cyclophosphamide by inhibiting its conversion to the active metabolite (Dixon, 1968).

Isoniazid is inactivated by genetically determined acetylation reactions. Patients who metabolize isoniazid slowly are more likely to become intoxicated when given phenytoin. This reaction is believed to be due to the higher concentrations of isoniazid in these individuals (Brennan *et al.*, 1970).

Excretion

Renal excretion of drugs depends upon glomerular filtration, tubular absorption and secretion, and non-ionic diffusion. Agents which alter renal blood flow also affect renal excretion. Glomerular filtration of drugs is mainly limited to the free or non-protein-bound fraction. Thus, agents which compete for serum protein binding sites (Tables IV and V) increase the proportion of free drug in the serum and increase renal clearance.

Drugs which interfere with tubular secretion exert the most profound effect on renal excretion (Table VIII). Probenecid is the prototype of these drugs. It is important to emphasize that probenecid will delay excretion, and thus, increase both blood levels and persistence of both penicillins and cephalosporins. Tubular secretion is so effective that even highly protein-bound penicillins which tend to exhibit lower glomerular filtration are rapidly cleared from the body.

TABLE VIII.

Decreased renal excretion of antimicrobial agents by other drugs.

Antibiotic	Other drug	Mechanism
Penicillins Cephalosporins Dapsone Nitrofurantoin	Probenecid Sulphaphenazole Sulphinpyrazone Acetylsalicylic acid	Competition for proximal tubular active transport
Cephaloridine	Furosemide	Unknown
Nitrofurantoin	Urinary acidification	Non-ionic diffusion

Most antimicrobial agents are weak acids (penicillins, cephalosporins, tetracyclines, sulphonamides, nitrofurantoin). These agents tend to be un-ionized at acid pH. At low rates of urine flow, they tend to diffuse back across the tubular cells. This in turn reduces renal clearance (Whelton and Walker, 1974). The reverse phenomenon is observed with weak bases (trimethoprim and erythromycin). Tubular uptake of aminoglycosides is more complex since these agents are highly polar and do not readily enter cells. Absorption of aminoglycosides by the proximal renal tubules is beyond the scope of this review.

Renal excretion of nitrofurantoin illustrates the complex roles of glomerular filtration, tubular secretion, and non-ionic diffusion (Schirmeister *et al.*, 1966). Nitrofurantoin is 60% protein-bound and the free proportion is filtered by the glomerulus. Most of the drug is secreted by the proximal renal tubule and may be blocked by *p*-aminohippuric acid and sulphinpyrazone.

Diuretic agents and antibiotics are often used simultaneously. Tice *et al.* (1975) demonstrated that the halflife of cephalothin in serum and urine was not significantly influenced by simultaneous administration of furosemide, mercaptomerin, and mannitol, or when no diuretic was given. In contrast, cephaloridine's halflife in serum was prolonged by moderate oral doses of furosemide (Norrby *et al.*, 1976). The mechanism of this interaction is unknown.

Direct Interaction

Interaction between aminoglycoside antibiotics which contain four or five free amino groups and carbenicillin and ticarcillin which possess two carboxyl groups has been described by many groups (Table IX). Amikacin appears to be less inhibited than gentamicin, tobramycin, and sisomicin (Holt *et al.*, 1976). Other penicillins and cephalosporins may inactivate aminoglycosides *in vitro*, but intravenous infusions or serum concentrations are too low to exert any major effect (Noone and Pattison, 1971). Most investigators agree that the interaction between these groups of antibiotics is not clinically significant, except in patients with

TABLE IX.

Direct antibiotic–drug interactions.

Antibiotic	Other drug	Interaction	Mechanism
Aminoglycosides	Carbenicillin	Aminoglycoside inactivation	Chemical interaction
	Ticarcillin	(clinically significant only in renal failure)	(β-lactam ring dependent)
Gentamicin	Heparin	Gentamicin activity decreased (not clinically significant *in vivo*)	Probably form complexes

severe renal failure (Davies *et al.*, 1975; Riff and Jackson, 1972). The kinetics of the interaction were studied in detail in patients with chronic renal failure by Ervin *et al.* (1976). They found overall reductions of gentamicin halflife in serum from 33 to 23 h with ticarcillin and from 46 to 22 h with carbenicillin.

Heparin, a negatively charged polyanion, combines with aminoglycoside antibiotics and tends to inactivate them. Regamey *et al.* (1972) demonstrated a reduction in gentamicin activity when the antibiotic was collected in heparinized tubes. This effect is unlikely to occur *in vivo* since serum levels of heparin needed for anticoagulation are well below the inhibitory concentrations exhibited *in vitro*.

CONCLUDING REMARKS

Antimicrobial agents exhibit potent pharmacologic effects in addition to their specific chemotherapeutic actions. Their disposition can be affected if they interact with other drugs, interfering with the optimum therapy for a patient. The simplest method to avoid these interactions is to use the minimum number of agents needed by the patient. Unforeseen interactions may occur, particularly when open orders for drugs such as sedatives, analgesics, and antacids, are given. Intravenous administration of fluids to adjust electrolyte balance may influence urinary pH and flow rates, and thus, affect renal handling of drugs. It is hoped that this review will be of help in alerting physicians to the problems that may be encountered in polypharmaceutical therapy.

ACKNOWLEDGEMENTS

We wish to thank Ms Cynthia Birch for editorial assistance in the preparation of this manuscript. This research was supported in part by the Medical Research Service of the Veterans Administration.

REFERENCES

General

Brodie, B. B. (1965). Displacement of one drug by another from carrier or receptor sites. *Proceedings of the Royal Society of Medicine* **58,** 946–955.

Burns, J. J. and Conney, A. H. (1965). Enzyme stimulation and inhibition in the metabolism of drugs. *Proceedings of the Royal Society of Medicine* **58,** 955–960.

Kabins, S. A. (1972). Interactions among antibiotics and other drugs. *Journal of the American Medical Association* **219,** 206–212.

Levy, G. (1976). Pharmacokinetic approaches to the study of drug interactions. *Annals of the New York Academy of Sciences* **281,** 24–39.

Prescott, L. F. (1969). Pharmacokinetic drug interactions. *Lancet* **ii,** 1239–1243.

Riley, H. D. (1972). Drug interactions—Part IV: Interactions among antimicrobial and nonantimicrobial agents. *Pediatrics* **50,** 954–955.

Absorption

Barr, W. H., Adir, J. and Garretson, L. (1971). Decrease of tetracycline absorption in man by sodium bicarbonate. *Clinical Pharmacology and Therapeutics* **12,** 779–784.

Boman, G. (1974). Serum concentration and half-life of rifampicin after simultaneous oral administration of aminosalicyclic acid or isoniazid. *European Journal of Clinical Pharmacology* **7,** 217–225.

Boman, G., Hanngren, Å., Malmrog, A., Borgå, O., ánd Sjögvist, F. (1971). Drug interaction: decreased serum concentrations of rifampicin when given with P.A.S. *Lancet* **1,** 800.

Boman, G., Lundgren, P. and Stjerström, G. (1975). Mechanism of the inhibitory effect of PAS granules on the absorption of rifampicin by an excipient, Bentonite. *European Journal of Clinical Pharmacology* **8,** 293–299.

Busfield, D., Child, K. J., Atkinson, R. M. and Tomich, E. G. (1963). An effect of phenobarbitone on blood levels of griseofulvin in man. *Lancet* **ii,** 1042–1043.

Cheng, S. H. and White, A. (1962). Effect of orally administered neomycin on the absorption of penicillin V. *New England Journal of Medicine* **267,** 1296–1297.

Fairfax, A. J., Adam, J. and Pagan, F. S. (1978). Effect of cimetidine on absorption of oral benzylpenicillin. *British Journal of Medicine* **1,** 820.

Gothoni, G., Pentikäinen, P., Vapaatalo, H. I., Hackman, R. and Björksten, K. A. F. (1972). Influence of metoclopramide and atropine on serum levels of pivampicillin and tetracycline. *Annals of Clinical Research* **4,** 228–232.

Gothoni, G., Neuvonen, P. J., Mattilia, M. and Hackman, R. (1972). Iron-tetracycline interaction: Effect of time interval between the drugs. *Acta Medica Scandinavica and Supplements* **191,** 409–411.

Greenberger, N. J., Ruppert, R. D. and Cuppage, F. E. (1967). Inhibition of intestinal iron transport induced by tetracycline. *Gastroenterology* **53,** 590–599.

Harcourt, R. S. and Hamburger, M. (1957). The effect of magnesium sulfate in lowering tetracycline blood levels. *Journal of Laboratory and Clinical Medicine* **50,** 464–468.

Lindenbaum, J., Maulitz, R. M. and Butler, V. P. (1976). Inhibition of digoxin absorption by neomycin. *Gastroenterology* **71,** 399–404.

Neuvonen, P. J. (1976). Interactions with the absorption of tetracyclines. *Drugs* **11,** 45–54.

Neuvonen, P. J., Gothoni, G., Hackman, R. and Björksten, K. A. F. (1970). Interference of iron with the absorption of tetracyclines in man. *British Medical Journal* **4,** 532–534.

Neuvonen, P. J. and Penttilä, O. (1974). Effect of oral ferrous sulphate on the half-life of doxycycline in man. *European Journal of Clinical Pharmacology* **7,** 361–363.

Neuvonen, P. J. and Turakka, H. (1974). Inhibitory effect of various iron salts on the absorption of tetracycline in man. *European Journal of Clinical Pharmacology* **7,** 357–360.

Penttilä, O., Hurme, H. and Neuvonen, P. J. (1975). Effect of zinc sulphate on the absorption of tetracycline and doxycycline in man. *European Journal of Clinical Pharmacology* **9,** 131–134.

Riegelman, S., Rowland, M. and Epstein, W. L. (1970). Griseofulvin–phenobarbital interaction in man. *Journal of the American Medical Association* **213,** 426–431.

Distribution

Anton, A. H. (1968). The effect of disease, drugs, and dilution on the binding of sulfonamides in human plasma. *Clinical Pharmacology and Therapeutics* **9,** 561–567.

Anton, A. H. (1960). The relation between the binding of sulfonamides to albumin and their antibacterial efficacy. *Journal of Pharmacology and Experimental Therapeutics* **129,** 282–290.

Anton, A. H. and Rodriguez, R. E. (1973). Drug-induced change in the distribution of sulfonamides in the mother rat and its fetus. *Science (N.Y.)* **180,** 974–976.

Christensen, L. K., Hansen, J. M. and Kristensen, M. (1963). Sulphaphenazole-induced hypoglycaemic attacks in tolbutamide-treated diabetics. *Lancet* **ii,** 1298–1301.

Craig, W. A. and Kunin, C. M. (1976). Significance of serum protein and tissue binding of antimicrobial agents. *Annual Review of Medicine* **27,** 287–300.

Dixon, R. L., Henderson, E. S. and Rail, D. P. (1965). Plasma protein binding of methotrexate and its displacement by various drugs. (Abstract No. 1807) *Federation Proceedings* **24,** 454.

Gibaldi, M. and Schwartz, M. A. (1968). Apparent effect of probenecid on the distribution of penicillins in man. *Clinical Pharmacology and Therapeutics* **9,** 345–349.

Kampmann, J., Hansen, J. M., Siersbaek-Nielsen, K. and Laursen, H. (1972). Effect of some drugs on penicillin half-life in blood. *Clinical Pharmacology and Therapeutics* **13,** 516–519.

Koch-Weser, J. and Sellers, E. M. (1976). Competition between drugs for albumin binding. (Second of two parts.) *New England Journal of Medicine* **294,** 526–531.

Kunin, C. M. (1966). Clinical pharmacology of the new penicillins: the importance of serum protein binding in determining antimicrobial activity and concentration in serum. *Clinical Pharmacology and Therapeutics* **7,** 166–179.

Kunin, C. M. (1966). Clinical pharmacology of the new penicillins: effect of drugs which interfere with binding to serum proteins. *Clinical Pharmacology and Therapeutics* **7,** 180–188.

Kunin, C. M. (1964). Enhancement of antimicrobial activity of penicillins and other antibiotics in human serum by competitive serum binding inhibitors. *Proceedings of the Society of Experimental Biology and Medicine* **117,** 69–73.

Moskowitz, B., Somani, S. M. and McDonald, R. H. (1973). Salicylate interaction with penicillin and secobarbital binding sites on human serum albumin. *Clinical Toxicology* **6,** 247–256.

Rolinson, R. N. and Sutherland, R. (1965). The binding of antibiotics of serum proteins. *British Journal of Pharmacology and Chemotherapy* **25,** 638–650.

Sellers, E. M. and Koch-Weser, J. (1970). Displacement of warfarin from human albumin by diazoxide and ethacrynic, mefenamic, and nalidixic acids. *Clinical Pharmacology and Therapeutics* **11,** 524–529.

Metabolism

Ballek, R. E., Reidenber, M. M. and Orr, L. (1973). Inhibition of diphenylhydantoin metabolism by chloramphenicol. *Lancet* **i,** 150.

Brennan, R. W., Dehejia, H., Kutt, H., Verebely, K. and McDowell, F. (1970). Diphenylhydantoin intoxication attendant to slow inactivation of isoniazid. *Neurology* **20,** 687–693.

Christensen, L. K. and Skovsted, L. (1969). Inhibition of drug metabolism by chloramphenicol. *Lancet* **ii,** 1397–1399.

Cullen, S. I. and Catalano, P. H. (1967). Griseofulvin-warfarin antagonism. *Journal of the American Medical Association* **199,** 150–151.

Dixon, R. L. (1968). Effect of chloramphenicol in the metabolism and lethality of cyclophosphamide in rats. *Proceedings of the Society of Experimental Biology and Medicine* **127,** 1151–1155.

Edwards, W. M., Galley, J. M., Courtenay-Evans, R. J., Hunter, J. and Tait, A. P. (1974). Changes in cortisol metabolism following rifampicin therapy. *Lancet* **ii,** 549–551.

Fallon, R. J., Allan, G. W., Lees, A. W., Smith, J. and Tyrrell, W. F. (1975). Probenecid and rifampicin serum levels. *Lancet* **ii,** 792–794.

Hempel, E. and Klinger, W. (1976). Drug-stimulated biotransformation of hormonal steroid contraceptives: clinical implications. *Drugs* **12,** 442–448.

Johnson, J. (1975). Epanutin and isoniazid interaction. *British Medical Journal* **1,** 152.

Kenwright, S. and Levi, A. J. (1973). Impairment of hepatic uptake of rifamycin antibiotics by probenecid, and its therapeutic implications. *Lancet* **ii,** 1402–1405.

Kreek, M. J., Garfield, J. W., Gutjahr, C. L. and Giusti, L. M. (1976). Rifampin-induced methadone withdrawal. *New England Journal of Medicine* **294,** 1104–1106.

Kutt, H., Brennan, R., Dehejia, H. and Verebely, K. (1970). Diphenylhydantoin intoxication: a complication of isoniazid therapy. *American Review of Respiratory Diseases* **101,** 377–384.

Llorens, J., Serrano, R. J. and Sanchez, R. (1978). Pharmacodynamic interference between rifampicin and isoniazid. *Chemotherapy* **24,** 97–103.

Neuvonen, P. J. and Penttilä, O. (1974). Interaction between doxycycline and barbiturates. *British Medical Journal* **1,** 535–536.

O'Reilly, R. A. (1975). Interaction of chronic daily warfarin therapy and rifampin. *Annals of Internal Medicine* **83,** 506–508.

O'Reilly, R. A. (1974). Interaction of sodium warfarin and rifampin. *Annals of Internal Medicine* **81,** 337–340.

Penttilä, O., Neuvonen, P. J., Aho, K. and Lehtovaara, R. (1974). Interaction between doxycycline and some antiepileptic drugs. *British Medical Journal* **2,** 470–472.

Radner, D. B. (1973). Toxicologic and pharmacologic aspects of rifampin. *Chest* **64,** 213–216.

Romankiewicz, J. A. and Ehrman, M. (1975). Rifampin and warfarin: a drug interaction. *Annals of Internal Medicine* **82,** 224–225.

Rose, J. Q., Choi, H. K., Schentag, J. J., Kinkel, W. R. and Jusko, W. J. (1977). Intoxication caused by interaction of chloramphenicol and phenytoin. *Journal of the American Medical Association* **237,** 2630–2631.

Self, T. H. and Mann, R. B. (1975). Interaction of rifampin and warfarin. *Chest* **67,** 490–491.

Tikkanen, M. J., Adlercreutz, H. and Pulkkinen, M. O. (1973). Effects of antibiotics on oestrogen metabolism. *British Medical Journal* **2,** 369.

Venho, V. M. K. and Koskinen, R. (1971). The effect of pyrazinamide, rifampicin and cycloserine on the blood levels and urinary excretion of isoniazid. *Annals of Clinical Research* **3,** 277–280.

Weinberger, M. (1978). Interaction between erythromycin and theophylline. *Pediatrics* **61,** 324–325. (Letter to the editor) Reply: Kozak, P. P., Cummin, L. H. and Gillman, S. A.

Excretion

Goodwin, C. S. and Sparell, G. (1969). Inhibition of dapsone excretion by probenecid. *Lancet* **ii,** 884–885.

Liegler, D. G., Henderson, E. S., Hahn, M. A. and Oliverio, V. T. (1969). The effect of organic acids on renal clearance of methotrexate in man. *Clinical Pharmacology and Therapeutics* **10,** 849–857.

Schirmeister, J., Stefani, F., Willman, H. and Hallover, W. (1966). Renal handling of nitrofurantoin in man. *In* "Antimicrobial Agents and Chemotherapy—1965", 223–226. American Society of Microbiology, Washington, D.C.

Tice, A. D., Barza, M., Bergeron, M. G., Brusch, J. L. and Weinstein, L. (1975). Effect of diuretics on urinary excretion of cephalothin in humans. *Antimicrobial Agents and Chemotherapy* **7,** 168–171.

Whelton, A. and Walker, W. G. (1974). Intrarenal antibiotic distribution in health and disease. *Kidney International* **6,** 131–137.

Direct Interactions

Davies, M., Morgan, J. R. and Anand, C. (1975). Interactions of carbenicillin and ticarcillin with gentamicin. *Antimicrobial Agents and Chemotherapy* **7,** 431–434.

Ervin, F. R., Bullock, W. E. and Nuttall, C. E. (1976). Inactivation of gentamicin by penicillins in patients with renal failure. *Antimicrobial Agents and Chemotherapy* **9,** 1004–1011.

Fillastre, J. P., Laumonier, R., Humbert, G., Dubois, D., Metayer, J., Delpech, A., Leroy, J. and Robert, M. (1973). Acute renal failure associated with combined gentamicin and cephalothin therapy. *British Medical Journal* **2,** 396–397.

Holt, H. A., Broughall, J. M., McCarthy, M. and Reeves, D. S. (1976). Interactions between aminoglycoside antibiotics and carbenicillin or ticarcillin. *Infection* **4,** 107–109.

McLaughlin, J. E. and Reeves, D. S. (1971). Clinical and laboratory evidence for inactivation of gentamicin by carbenicillin. *Lancet* **i,** 261–264.

Noone, P. and Pattison, J. R. (1971). Therapeutic implications of interaction of gentamicin and penicillins. *Lancet* **i,** 575–578.

Norrby, R., Stenqvist, K. and Elgefors, B. (1976). Interaction between cephaloridine and furosemide in man. *Scandinavian Journal of Infectious Diseases* **8,** 209–212.

Regamey, C., Schaberg, D. and Kirby, W. M. (1972). Inhibitory effect of heparin on gentamicin concentrations in blood. *Antimicrobial Agents and Chemotherapy* **1,** 329–332.

Riff, L. J. and Jackson, G. G. (1972). Laboratory and clinical conditions for gentamicin inactivation by carbenicillin. *Archives of Internal Medicine* **130,** 887–891.

Weibert, R., Keane, W. and Shapiro F. (1976). Carbenicillin inactivation of aminoglycosides in patients with severe renal failure. *Transactions; American Society for Artificial Internal Organs* **22,** 439–443.

Weibert, R. T. and Keane, W. F. (1977). Carbenicillin–gentamicin interaction in acute renal failure. *American Journal of Hospital Pharmacists* **34,** 1137–1139.

DISCUSSION

O'Grady Can we take it overall that as far as the antibiotic side is concerned there are no problems? This is to say that interactions are such that the activity of the antibiotic is not compromised?

Kunin There are many instances where the activity of the antimicrobial agent might be compromised as pointed out in my review of the literature. In most instances, however, these effects would probably not interfere with effective chemotherapy since the dosage schedules we commonly use to treat infectious diseases are often more than adequate. I can visualize situations, however, where interactions with other agents combined with problems of compliance, absorption, underlying disease, and so forth, might lead to inadequate therapy.

Asscher Another category of interaction seen with antibacterial agents happens in the laboratory. Nalidixic acid, for instance, interferes with urinary vanillyl mandelic acid estimation and this may lead to the erroneous diagnosis of phaeochromocytoma. Trimethoprim may interfere with the tubular secretion of creatinine which occurs in patients with kidney failure and so produce reduction of creatinine clearance which is not paralleled by a reduction of glomerular filtration. I suspect Professor Kunin had quite enough interactions to relate to us to allow him to include these in-vitro interactions, yet they can seriously mislead clinicians.

Brumfitt Did you say that during the administration of rifampicin and trimethoprim after seven days the trimethoprim halflife falls to 80% of its usual value, I wonder if you could tell me why?

TABLE I.

Mean urine concentrations of rifampicin (R) and trimethoprim (T) in five patients given 600 mg R + 160 mg T daily at bedtime.

	Concentrations (μg ml^{-1}) at indicated collection periods (hours)							Recovery (%) at indicated periods (hours)	
	0–12	12–14	14–16	16–18	18–20	20–22	22–24	0–12	12–24
Rifampicin									
Day 1	189	126	112	74·2	33·8	26·8	19·0	31·7	6·0
Day 7	347	12·2	11·0	6·43	2·74	1·60	1·41	26·9	0·5
Trimethoprim									
Day 1	117	82·7	75·0	70·7	44·4	59·2	33·7	37·3	19·1
Day 7	159	50·2	31·8	27·6	17·7	13·7	17·3	44·0	9·5

Kosmidis Perhaps I can give you some information in this respect. In the study I mentioned before, we measured the amount of drugs recovered in urine every two hours for 24 hours in some of the patients receiving rifaprim once daily. This was done on the first and seventh day. It was shown that although the total amount of trimethoprim recovered in 24 hours was not much lowered in the seventh day, 53·5% compared to 56·4% during the first day, there was a shift of a considerable size from the second 12-hour period to the first such period: 37·3% of dose was recovered in the first 12 hours and 19·1% in the second 12 hours on the first day, while on the seventh day recovery reached 44% in the first 12 hours and only 9·5% in the second 12 hours (Table I). These results imply that there might have been a quicker excretion via the kidney.

Kunin Dr Kosmidis, would you please clarify whether your chemical assay distinguishes between biologically active trimethoprim versus inactive or less active metabolites?

Kosmidis I used a biological assay.

Kunin Yes, they did test different forms of Warfarin.

Percival There is also interaction when a drug is inactivated by conjugation in the liver but thereafter partially or totally deconjugated by gut flora and recycled by reabsorption. Suppression of gut flora by antimicrobials may then diminish the effectiveness of the other drug because deconjugation and recycling are reduced. For example, antimicrobials may thus interfere with oral contraceptives. We have recently shown interference of the enterohepatic circulation by steroids in rats; partially by neomycin which does not reduce anaerobes, more completely by ampicillin or neomycin plus lincomycin but hardly at all by rifampicin because of rapid emergence of a resistant faecal flora. However, an antibiotic such as rifampicin could reduce the effectiveness of another drug by inductive stimulation of conjugating liver enzymes.

Kunin To expand on the point brought out by Dr Percival regarding activity of antibiotics on the gut, I would like to point out the following. Antibiotics in themselves do not necessarily decrease enzymatic activity of microorganisms. Urease, for example, is not affected by neomycin. Urease production in the gut is decreased by neomycin only because it inhibits bacterial growth after the bacteria are shed in the faeces.

Brumfitt One of the major problems is the difficulty in estimating the excretion of these compounds in the bile. Techniques are now becoming available but excretion of antibiotics in the bile is not constant; it is intermittent and variable. Nevertheless, I think too little effort has been made to study the rate of flow, or excretion.

Cole I would like to comment on the gentamicin–carbenicillin interaction. It is always said that the penicillin is inactivating the aminoglycoside. In regard to the chemistry of the reaction you referred to the fact that the β-lactam ring had to be intact. We examined what happened the other way round and we found that the aminoglycoside would rapidly inactivate the penicillin. If you put them together in a one-to-one mixture you find they are both being inactivated. What is happening is that the β-lactam ring is acylating an amino group on the aminoglycoside so that the two molecules are reacting—possible in the one-to-one ratio—to give you an inactive aminoglycoside and an inactive penicillin.

Kunin This explanation is quite helpful to me. I must confess that I thought that only the carboxyl groups of the penicillins were involved in the reaction.

Jackson I can confirm what Dr Cole said (see Perenyi *et al.*, 1974). The gentamicin activity, however, can be reconstituted by a reducing agent, perhaps causing deacylation. But you cannot reconstitute the β-lactam ring. One activity is clinically and microbiologically important because on a molecular basis the inactivation in a one-to-one ratio decreases the amount of gentamicin that is biologically effective whereas if you take out a few molecules of penicillin it is not important. The chemistry is that of mutual inactivation but the biological effect is greater.

Brumfitt Are the interesting studies described by Dr Kunin carried out in man? I have in mind the fact that the halflife of trimethoprim in the human is 8–10 hours and in the mouse one hour.

Kunin Most of the studies reported in my review were done in humans.

Brumfitt I am frightened of animal studies as a basis of discussing interactions.

Kunin I was not extrapolating from animal studies. I didn't really need to since I had to screen through about 2000 records of drug interactions in man.

Jackson In your initial remarks, Mr Chairman, you said we can assume that none of these drug-inactivating reactions have clinical importance in terms of the antibiotic effect. I wanted to have Dr Kunin respond to that because I am not entirely easy with that summary conclusion.

It seems to me there are two questions: one is drug inactivation in the absorptive phase; the other is the chemical interaction such as with gentamicin and β-lactam drugs where the clearance times are so delayed that in-vivo inactivation can occur—for example in uraemic patients, or in joint fluids, the cerebrospinal fluid and perhaps other fluid collections in which the pharmacokinetics permit a longer time for inactivation of the same molecules.

Kunin This is a major reason for keeping chemotherapy simple. The less often we use multiple drugs at the same time in a given patient, the less we have to be concerned about unsuspected interactions.

Jackson Is the Chairman correct in minimizing antibiotic interactions?

Kunin My response is to keep chemotherapy as simple as possible. We can, however, anticipate problems by analysing which drugs are commonly given together. From such a profile we could predict which group of patients suffering from a specific disease (and therefore receiving certain agents) would be at highest risk of interaction when antimicrobial agents are added to their treatment.

Black The number of side-effects and interactions of drugs is so vast that they would over-saturate the binding sites of our memories. We must therefore welcome (and use) mechanical aids such as the Goldberg disc. Even so, we run into trouble when, as may happen, the same patient is being treated by more than one doctor.

Lambert The problem of enzyme induction by rifampicin may be encountered quite commonly. We have seen three patients whose Addison's disease became manifest or deteriorated because of increased steroid requirement following rifampicin therapy for pulmonary or meningeal tuberculosis.

REFERENCE

Perenyi, T., Graber, H. and Arr, M. (1974). Über die Wechselwirkung der Penizilline und aminoglycosid antibiotika. *International Journal of Clinical Pharmacology, Therapy and Toxicology* **10,** 50–55.

Laboratory Methods for the Evaluation of Synergy

DAVID GREENWOOD

Department of Microbiology, University Hospital,
Queen's Medical Centre, Nottingham, UK.

The basic methods by which the interaction of antibacterial compounds may be demonstrated in the laboratory and the interpretation of such interactions in clinical terms has been exhaustively dealt with on numerous occasions during the last thirty years, notably by the doyen of combination studies, Ernest Jawetz (Jawetz, 1952, 1968a, b, 1975). The subject has, in fact, held a peculiar fascination for microbiologists ever since the possibility existed of mixing two antibacterial substances in a test-tube; being a fundamentally optimistic group of people, they have generally carried out their studies in the hope or expectation of achieving an enhanced—that is synergic—effect.

While I should like to continue this optimistic tradition by concentrating mainly on synergic aspects of antibacterial interactions, there seems little point in reiterating what has been said so often and so well before. Consequently, I intend in this paper to consider some aspects of synergy which seem to have received less attention. The first and foremost of these is the diversity of form which synergic interactions can take, an understanding of which is fundamental to any attempt to demonstrate or evaluate synergy in the laboratory.

TYPES OF SYNERGY

Known synergic interactions between antibacterial agents can generally be placed into four broad categories, which may be further subdivided on the basis of different modes of antibacterial action (Table I). It can be seen from the table that β-lactam antibiotics—penicillins and cephalosporins—provide examples of each of the different broad groups. This family of antibiotics appears to be particularly rich in synergic potential, displaying clear examples of synergy between members of the group as well as with unrelated antibacterial agents. A consideration of

TABLE I.
Types of synergy.

Type	Mechanism	Drugs
Biochemical interaction	sequential blockade complementation	trimethoprim–sulphonamides mecillinam–cephalexin
Permeabilization	cell wall cell membrane	β-lactam antibiotics polymyxins
Protection	β-lactamase inhibition	nafcillin, clavulanic acid
Differential population effects	suppression of resistance	antituberculosis therapy: penicillin–fusidic acid, rifampicin–nalidixic acid

TABLE II.
Examples of synergy involving β-lactam antibiotics.

Type of synergy	Bacteria chiefly affected	Example of effective combination
β-Lactamase inhibition	gram-negative bacilli	clavulanic acid– broad-spectrum β-lactams
Complementation	gram-negative bacilli	cephalexin–mecillinam
Lysis enhancement	gram-negative bacilli	cephalexin–cephalothin
Dual activity	gram-negative bacilli	omadine–cephalosporin (Glaxo compound MCO)
Permeabilization	enterococci, etc. gram-negative bacilli	penicillins–aminoglycosides ampicillin–erythromycin
Mutual suppression of resistance	staphylococci	penicillin–fusidic acid

some of the synergic interactions in which β-lactam antibiotics are involved (Table II) will therefore serve to highlight the plurality of synergic phenomena.

β-lactamase Inhibition

This is the most familiar form of synergy occurring between β-lactam antibiotics. It depends on the fact that resistance to β-lactam antibiotics is generally due to the production of antibiotic-destroying enzymes which can be inhibited by one β-lactam compound (which need have no antibacterial activity in its own right), thus protecting a more susceptible, but antibacterially active compound from destruction. Interest in this concept has received new impetus from the discovery of clavulanic acid, a naturally occurring compound produced by *Streptomyces clavuligerus*, which is an unusually potent, broad-spectrum inhibitor (Reading and Cole, 1977).

Complementation

Like trimethoprim–sulphonamide synergy, this is a form of double blockade in which two antibiotics act at different, but related sites, in this case in the bacterial cell wall. Complementation is displayed between cephalosporins of the cephalexin type (cephalexin, cephradine, cephaloglycin) which induce filamentation in gram-negative bacilli by interfering with a particular protein involved in cell division (Spratt, 1975) and certain β-lactam antibiotics, of which mecillinam is the best known example, which act against a different protein (Spratt, 1975), and elicit different morphological changes (Greenwood and O'Grady, 1973a). In combination cephalexin and mecillinam complement one another to produce, in gram-negative bacilli, the spheroplast response typically induced by high concentrations of most other β-lactam agents which act at both sites (Greenwood and O'Grady, 1973b).

Lysis Enhancement

This is a special form of the complementation effect which also depends on the unusual filament forming behaviour of cephalexin-like compounds. Most β-lactam antibiotics, at concentrations somewhat above the minimum inhibitory concentration, induce rapid lysis in susceptible gram-negative bacilli. In the presence of agents of the cephalexin type, the concentration of other β-lactam antibiotics required to cause lysis of gram-negative bacilli is considerably reduced (Greenwood and O'Grady, 1975). A further reduction is observed if the bacteria are pre-exposed to the filament inducer, and the phenomenon is no doubt due to residual lytic activity of the second agent being apparently enhanced by being directed against non-septate filaments instead of normal-sized bacteria.

Dual Activity

This is an ingenious manoeuvre for bolstering the activity of cephalosporins, which often have only a transient lytic effect on bacteria because the antibiotic is broken down enzymically and regrowth of persisting bacteria occurs. The stratagem consists in linking a second antibacterial compound to a cephalosporin at the 3-position of the cephem nucleus. The prototype molecule of this kind is the Glaxo compound MCO (O'Callaghan *et al.*, 1976; Greenwood and O'Grady, 1976a) in which 2-mercaptopyridine-*N*-oxide (omadine) is linked to α-hydroxyphenylacetamidocephalosporanic acid. The entire molecule behaves like a cephalosporin and can, in suitable circumstances, cause rapid bacterial lysis. If the compound is attacked by *β*-lactamases, however, the antibacterial substituent, omadine, is released to prolong the antibacterial activity.

Permeabilization

This is the classic form of interaction between penicillins and aminoglycosides against enterococci, although many other bacteria are affected in a similar way. What appears to happen is that sub-lethal concentrations of penicillin cause sufficient cell wall damage to allow the aminoglycoside (which is normally excluded) into the cell. The end result is that a more rapid bactericidal effect is achieved by the mixture than by either of the components. A somewhat analagous situation arises when erythromycin (normally excluded from coliform bacilli) is used to inhibit *β*-lactam-induced spheroplasts—cell wall deficient forms of gram-negative bacilli. In this case, the principle will only operate if the osmolality of the environment is sufficiently high to allow spheroplasts to survive (Greenwood and O'Grady, 1972), otherwise these osmotically fragile forms will lyse and the erythromycin will have no function to perform.

Mutual Suppression of Resistance

Use of combinations of antibiotics mutually to suppress resistant minority populations is a concept generally thought of in the context of antituberculosis therapy, but can also be applied to other bacterial infections. Thus penicillin and fusidic acid may be used in this way against penicillinase-producing staphylococci on the basis that most of the staphylococci are dealt with by the fusidic acid while fusidic acid-resistant mutants are mopped up by the penicillin (Waterworth, 1963). An interesting sidelight on this particular combination is that penicillin and fusidic acid are mutually antagonistic against many strains of staphylococci (Mouton and Koelman, 1966). Against these strains, penicillin interferes with the bactericidal activity of fusidic acid by preventing the secondary cell wall collapse which appears to occur as a consequence of the inhibition of protein synthesis.

This unexpected effect is readily seen in the scanning electron microscope (O'Grady and Greenwood, 1973).

It is clear from this brief consideration of the multiple forms that synergy may take that no one laboratory test is going to reveal each kind, let alone help to evaluate its significance. Notwithstanding this, a handful of tests tend to be used indiscriminately, and often uncritically, when antimicrobial interactions are under study. The most commonly employed in-vitro method is the chessboard titration test. A consideration of the scope of this test and the type of information it generates will show that results obtained in this way need to be interpreted with some caution.

Chessboard Titrations

The results of chessboard titrations may be expressed in terms of changes in the minimum inhibitory concentrations (MICs) or minimum bactericidal concentrations (MBCs) of the interacting compounds. In practice, the additional labour of estimating the MBC is often dispensed with and the MIC results, expressed as the sum of the fractional inhibitory concentration (ΣFIC) of the components of the mixture taken as the measure of synergy.

While several of the types of interaction listed in Tables I and II may be detected in suitable circumstances by bactericidal chessboard tests (even better by constructing killing curves), only two—trimethoprim–sulphonamide synergy and β-lactamase inhibition—can be detected with any degree of confidence in chessboard titrations employing inhibitory criteria alone. Curiously, the β-lactamase inhibition type of synergy, on the basis of which spectacular isobolograms can be constructed, does not exhibit the form of interaction which chessboard titrations are intended to detect—a mutual enhancement of antibacterial potency—because the activity of the inhibitor is not, of course, influenced by the second, antibacterially active, compound.

Chessboard titrations, then, at least of the bacteriostatic variety, have a distinctly limited usefulness in the detection of the full range of antimicrobial interactions. That is not all, however. Even in cases where the technique seems to come into its own, for example in delineating the extent of synergy between trimethoprim and sulphonamides, the method has certain inherent weaknesses because of its reliance on the MIC end-point as the criterion of effectiveness.

Quite apart from the well-known variables (composition of medium, inoculum size, etc.) which may affect the result, MIC tests only record the end result of a series of events which have taken place during the incubation period (usually overnight—16 to 20 hours). In fact, the phrase "minimum inhibitory concentration", hallowed though it is by long microbiological usage and inexpedient to alter now, is a misnomer. All antibacterial agents have considerable inhibitory activity at concentrations below the so-called MIC and the factors which determine the ultimate end-point vary widely from one antibacterial agent to another (Greenwood, 1976). Polymyxin B, for example, at concentrations ranging from 1/32 to 1/2 MIC, selects out a series of phenotypic variants of increasing resistance and the end-point of MIC tests reflects the suppression of the most resistant of these. Similar sub-MIC levels of chloramphenicol, on the other hand, have a progressively greater effect on the growth rate of the whole bacterial population and the MIC end-point is the lowest concentration which succeeds in holding the population below the threshold of visibility throughout the period of incubation (Greenwood, 1976).

As chessboard titrations, by definition, employ sub-MIC antibiotic levels, the nature of events taking place at these levels is clearly likely to influence the final outcome of the test. In many cases (trimethoprim, sulphonamides, aminoglycosides, etc.), the MIC end-point is determined by the emergence, during the overnight incubation period, of variants which exhibit a small increment of resistance to the drug (Greenwood and O'Grady, 1976b; Mawer and Greenwood, 1978). In other words, the MIC is influenced by the ability of some bacteria in the population to adapt to otherwise inhibitory drug levels. When such drugs are combined at sub-MIC levels, one of the effects that is observed is that "adaptive" resistance is mutually suppressed. In the case of the trimethoprim–sulphonamide combination this effect, which is probably unrelated to the sequential blockade phenomenon, appears to be a substantial component of the overall synergy detected in chessboard titrations (Greenwood and O'Grady, 1976b; Greenwood, 1977).

In order to omit this component from the overall equation, synergy can be alternatively assessed on the basis of reductions in the minimum antibacterial concentration (MAC)—a term which has been coined to designate the lowest concentration causing an observable antibacterial effect, conveniently detected as a deviation from the normal growth curve by continuous turbidimetric monitoring. Viewed in this way, synergy between trimethoprim and sulphamethoxazole is still displayed, in that concentrations lower than the MAC of each component can combine to produce an antibacterial effect, but the degree of synergy is considerably reduced (Table III). In fact the extent of synergy detected using the MAC criterion is more in keeping with what one would predict on the basis of simple sequential blockade of a metabolic pathway.

IN-VITRO POINTERS TO THE CLINICAL SIGNIFICANCE OF SYNERGY

One of the chief complaints about in-vitro tests in general, and tests of synergy in particular, is that it is difficult to assess their meaning in clinical terms. The conditions in which antibacterial agents are expected to exert their effect in treat-

TABLE III.

Synergy between trimethoprim and sulphamethoxazole expressed in terms of the minimum antibacterial concentration and minimum inhibitory concentration.

Smallest concentration producing	
Deviation from normal growth	Suppression of growth overnight
TMP + SMX	TMP + SMX
MAC/2 + MAC/8	MIC/8 + MIC/32
MAC/4 + MAC/2	MIC/16 + MIC/8

TMP = trimethoprim; SMX = sulphamethoxazole;
MAC = minimum antibacterial concentration;
MIC = minimum inhibitory concentration.

ment are so different from those which prevail *in vitro* that meaningful statements are difficult to make. In the case of combination therapy there is the added difficulty that pharmacokinetic differences between antibiotics can lead to a situation where the two agents never meet in the body in the way they do in the test-tube.

Laboratory tests can be made more meaningful by arranging for bacterial cultures to be exposed to antibacterial agents in ways which approximate more closely to the in-vivo situation. A device which has proved useful in this way is an in-vitro model of the urinary bladder (Greenwood and O'Grady, 1978) in which a bacterial culture, maintained in a semicontinuous cultivation state, such as exists in infected urine, can be exposed to a changing drug concentration (in simulation of the renal excretion profile) by use of a gradient-forming device.

As a contribution to the debate as to whether trimethoprim should be used alone in the treatment of urinary tract infection, this model has been used to try to answer the question of whether trimethoprim–sulphamethoxazole synergy operates in the conditions existing during treatment in which concentrations of the two drugs well above the MIC are achievable for long periods. It turns out that, in the presence of levels of trimethoprim well within those achievable in urine on modest dosage, the sulphonamide component contributes nothing to the overall antibacterial effect (Greenwood, 1977; Greenwood and O'Grady, 1976b). Indeed, trimethoprim may be considered to antagonize sulphonamides: trimethoprim acts relatively quickly by trapping folic acid in the inactive dihydrofolate form, whereas sulphonamides prevent fresh folate being formed, and halt bacterial growth only after several generations because preformed folate continues to be utilized until continued growth and division dilute the pool to below a functional level. In the presence of sufficient trimethoprim bacterial growth is rapidly inhibited and the sulphonamide gets no opportunity to act.

Here, then, is an example of two antibacterial agents displaying outstanding synergy in chessboard titrations which is likely to be totally irrelevant in therapeutic terms, at least in those clinical situations in which supra-MIC concentrations can be reliably maintained. But the converse situation may also arise: failure to detect synergy in chessboard titrations may conceal a potentially useful combination. An example of this may be furnished by nalidixic acid and rifampicin. Both these agents are highly active against a wide range of microorganisms, but the effectiveness of both is mitigated to some extent by the ready emergence of resistant bacteria, both in the test-tube and the patient (Ronald, *et al.*, 1966; Finegold *et al.*, 1967; Atlas and Turck, 1968; McCabe and Lorian, 1968). There is scope, therefore, to apply the same principle as is used in antituberculosis therapy —to achieve a combined effect by the mutual suppression of resistant variants. The frequency with which resistant mutants are met increases markedly with the size of the bacterial population and synergy of this type may be detected in chessboard titrations only when dense inocula are used, in which case trailing end-points make the test difficult to read (Greenwood and Andrew, 1978).

Dense bacterial populations are frequently present in infection, however, and the behaviour of such populations in the presence of antibacterial agents may be relevant to the outcome of treatment. When nalidixic acid and rifampicin were tested against the dense bacterial population of the bladder model, it was found that nalidixic acid alone could suppress bacterial growth effectively, providing a high drug level was maintained, in agreement with the clinical observations of Stamey and Bragonje (1976); rifampicin alone was unable to suppress growth for long periods because of the emergence of resistance. These studies also revealed that high dosage of nalidixic acid was only necessary to accommodate the minority resistant population; in combination with rifampicin, long-term suppression of bacterial growth was achieved with much-reduced levels of the two agents (Table 4).

TABLE IV.

Suppression of bacterial growth in the bladder model by nalidixic acid and rifampicin, alone and in combination. (From Greenwood and Andrew, 1978.)

Antibacterial agent	Plateau level ($\mu g\ ml^{-1}$)	Time before growth detectable (h)
Nalidixic acid	50	22
Rifampicin	50	12
Nalidixic acid	2	
plus	+	>40
Rifampicin	10	

In an article in the *British Medical Journal* written 25 years ago, Professor Garrod, in considering laboratory methods, was led to state "Unfortunately, simple tests of growth inhibition, at least by pairs of antibiotics, seem to be worthless" (Garrod, 1953). Pessimism about using simple inhibitory criteria for detecting antimicrobial interactions is well founded. Even in those cases in which such tests suggest impressive synergy the clinical relevance of the results needs interpreting with great care, while too great a reliance on "chessboard synergy" may divert attention from therapeutically more useful forms of drug interaction.

REFERENCES

Atlas, E. and Turck, M. (1968). Laboratory and clinical evaluation of rifampicin. *American Journal of the Medical Sciences* **256,** 247–254.

Finegold, S. M., Miller, L. G., Posnick, D., Patterson, D. K. and Davis, A. (1967). Nalidixic acid: clinical and laboratory studies. *Antimicrobial Agents and Chemotherapy—*1966 179–189.

Garrod, L. P. (1953). Combined chemotherapy in bacterial infections. *British Medical Journal* **1,** 953–957.

Greenwood, D. (1976). Differentiation of mechanisms responsible for inoculum effects in the response of *Escherichia coli* to a variety of antibiotics. *Journal of Antimicrobial Chemotherapy* **2,** 87–95.

Greenwood, D. (1977). Trimethoprim plus sulphamethoxazole: synergic or antagonistic combination? *In* "Antibiotics and Antibiosis in Agriculture" (Ed. M. Woodbine), 82–88. Butterworths, London.

Greenwood, D. and Andrew, J. (1978). Rifampicin plus nalidixic acid: a rational combination for the treatment of urinary infection. *Journal of Antimicrobial Chemotherapy* **4,** 533–538.

Greenwood, D. and O'Grady, F. (1972). The effect of osmolality on the response of *Escherichia coli* and *Proteus mirabilis* to penicillins. *British Journal of Experimental Pathology* **53,** 457–464.

Greenwood, D. and O'Grady, F. (1973a). FL 1060: a new beta-lactam antibiotic with novel properties. *Journal of Clinical Pathology* **26,** 1–6.

Greenwood, D. and O'Grady, F. (1973b). The two sites of penicillin action in *Escherichia coli*. *Journal of Infectious Diseases* **128,** 791–794.

Greenwood, D. and O'Grady, F. (1975). Lysis enhancement: a novel form of interaction between *β*-lactam antibiotics. *Journal of Medical Microbiology* **8,** 105–108.

Greenwood, D. and O'Grady, F. (1976a). Dual-action cephalosporin utilizing a novel therapeutic principle. *Antimicrobial Agents and Chemotherapy* **10,** 249–252.

Greenwood, D. and O'Grady, F. (1976b). Activity and interaction of trimethoprim and sulphamethoxazole against *Escherichia coli*. *Journal of Clinical Pathology* **29,** 162–166.

Greenwood, D. and O'Grady, F. (1978). An in-vitro model of the urinary bladder. *Journal of Antimicrobial Chemotherapy* **4,** 113–120.

Jawetz, E. (1952). Antibiotic synergism and antagonism: a review of experimental evidence. *Archives of Internal Medicine* **90,** 301–309.

Jawetz, E. (1968a). Combined antibiotic action: some definitions and correlations between laboratory and clinical results. Antimicrobial Agents and Chemotherapy—1967. 203–209.

Jawetz, F. (1968b). The use of combinations of antimicrobial drugs. *Annual Review of Pharmacology* **8,** 151–170.

Jawetz, E. (1975). Actions of antimicrobial drugs in combination. *Veterinary Clinics of North America* **5,** 35–50.

Mawer, S. L. and Greenwood, D. (1978). Specific and non-specific resistance to aminoglycosides in *Escherichia coli*. *Journal of Clinical Pathology* **31,** 12–15.

McCabe, W. R. and Lorian, V. (1968). Comparison of the antibacterial activity of rifampicin and other antibiotics. *American Journal of the Medical Sciences* **256,** 255–265.

Mouton, R. P. and Koelman, A. (1966). The interaction patterns of combined antibacterial agents. *Chemotherapia* **11,** 10–26.

O'Callaghan, C. H., Sykes, R. B. and Staniforth, S. E. (1976). A new cephalosporin with a dual mode of action. *Antimicrobial Agents and Chemotherapy* **10,** 246–248.

O'Grady, F. and Greenwood, D. (1973). Interactions between fusidic acid and penicillins. *Journal of Medical Microbiology* **6,** 441–450.

Reading, C. and Cole, M. (1977). Clavulanic acid: a beta-lactamase-inhibiting beta-lactam from *Streptomyces clavuligerus*. *Antimicrobial Agents and Chemotherapy* **11,** 852–857.

Ronald, A. R., Turck, M. and Petersdorf, R. G. (1966). A critical evaluation of nalidixic acid in urinary-tract infection. *New England Journal of Medicine* **275,** 1081–1089.

Spratt, B. G. (1975). Distinct penicillin-binding proteins involved in the division, elongation and shape of *Escherichia coli* K12. *Proceedings of the National Academy of Sciences of the United States of America* **72,** 2999–3003.

Stamey, T. A. and Bragonje, J. (1976). Resistance to nalidixic acid, a misconception due to underdosage. *Journal of the American Medical Association* **236,** 1857–1860.

Waterworth, P. M. (1963). Apparent synergy between penicillin and erythromycin or fusidic acid. *Clinical Medicine* **70,** 941–953.

DISCUSSION

Black Some of your slides suggested that the ratio between two potentially synergistic agents might be important. One can control that in the laboratory, but if one then goes back to Dr Kunin's evidence it is clear that that ratio might be seriously distorted in treatment. Is it correct that the ratio is critical as well as the concentrations, and, if so, is this a further reason why the natural optimism of the microbiologist may not lead directly to clinical miracles?

Greenwood I don't think that the actual ratio is important. The ratio discussion came up first with cotrimoxazole and is a red herring which has obscured the real issue. With trimethoprim and sulphonamides synergy is simply inoperative—at least at the concentrations which are easily achievable in urine when the activity of trimethoprim completely swamps that of the sulphonamide. So, in urinary tract infection at least, the ratio doesn't matter at all. With nalidixic acid and rifampicin, I don't think the ratio matters either as long as the pharmacokinetics are roughly comparable. One is mutually preventing the emergence of resistance, so you need one agent to dispose of the majority of the bacteria, which are highly sensitive, and a little of the other to mop up resistant mutants which may emerge.

Kunin I am rather puzzled by this observation. I thought that in other models, trimethoprim and sulphamethoxazole had an action above and beyond what you described. They have been shown to be more bactericidal against many organisms alone than either component. Perhaps you would say a few words about this kind of synergy. I am particularly interested in their action in the kidney, not simply the bladder urine.

Greenwood With the urinary strains we use we have not been able to detect any bactericidal synergy with cotrimoxazole. This should be detectable in our system by an increase in the time taken for regrowth to occur: if two agents together are more bactericidal than the components it should take longer for survivors to re-emerge when the drugs are removed.

Kass I am concerned along similar lines. If we try to relate the in-vitro sensitivity pattern to the outcome of treatment of patients with urinary tract infection we must start with the realization that the organism will often be cleared by the urinary tract even without antibiotics. Why does your model fail to reflect what we know to be true clinically? Can we accept the lessons of a laboratory model if it doesn't seem to be coordinated with clinical responses?

When we examine the sensitivity of an organism to sulphonamides we limit ourselves to rather small inocula. They are difficult substances to test and laboratory results do not always reflect the therapeutic response that we do get. In your system you are working with turbidimetry which translated into actual numbers of bacteria operates from 4 or 5×10^7, up to 5 or 6×10^9. The initial inocula are so high that it is almost impossible to see any effect from sulphonamides so I am not surprised that you see very little difference between the combination and single agents. Will the experiments be repeated with much lower inocula? One really asks why sulphonamides are effective in the urinary tract, or elsewhere, when bacterial numbers are high.

Greenwood As regards the validity of the model, this is acknowledged to be a glass bladder in an incubator and not a bladder in any physiological sense but it does take us one step closer to the in-vivo situation. With antibacterial therapy, the proof is in clinical response but it is extremely difficult to get precise data from clinical trials, and to get meaningful comparative figures for cure rates in urinary tract infection is particularly difficult. Therefore, we need to examine either animals, which also have problems of interpretation or go back to the test-tube. The bladder model is a way of bringing the test-tube closer to reality. Mechanically at least it simulates the situation which exists in the bladder where the bacterial population is in a dynamic state and is exposed to concentrations of antibiotics that rise and fall as they do during therapy. That is the rationale; whether it has a bearing on the clinical situation only extensive clinical trials can show.

Your second point concerns sulphonamides and the inoculum effect. Here the bladder model has shown itself very useful in answering the very problem you raise: why, in urinary tract infection, where there is often a dense bacterial population, are sulphonamides therapeutically effective, whereas conventional laboratory tests suggest that sulphonamides have no activity against such large bacterial numbers? In the bladder model, as in the patient, sulphonamides have a very marked effect against dense bacterial populations because the model, like the human bladder, is a semicontinuous cultivation system: Sulphonamides do not inhibit growth until the bacterial folate pool is diluted out by continued growth and therefore bacteria exposed to sulphonamides continue to grow for several generations. In static test-tube systems the population achieves visible proportions (or if the initial inoculum is dense enough, enters the stationary phase) before any antibacterial effect is seen. In the bladder model, a semicontinuous culture system, one can suppress a very dense bacterial population with sub-MIC levels of sulphonamides.

Kunin If growth continues, how can the opacity show a downward shift?

Greenwood In the model the bacterial culture is being continuously diluted and periodically discharged. In these circumstances, as the folate pool becomes depleted, growth stops and the bacteria are washed away.

Kunin But the conclusion that I gathered was that the combination of trimethoprim and sulphamethoxazole probably will not work because it did not work in this system. That does not fit the facts.

Greenwood What the bladder model showed was that in the presence of sufficient trimethoprim the sulphonamide had no *additional* effect. In trying to answer the question: "Does synergy operate at the supra-MIC levels that are achieved during therapy?" The answer I have come up with is: "No, it doesn't". Furthermore, there are good theoretical reasons why synergy should not operate in these circumstances.

Smith Another thing that causes confusion with sulphonamide and also with trimethoprim or nalidixic acid, is that the bacteria can be dying rapidly while the actual opacity of the culture is increasing. This occurs because the dying bacteria elongate to form filaments. So if opacity measurements alone are recorded the data give completely the opposite picture to what is actually happening.

I quite agree that sulphonamide cannot improve anything that trimethoprim can do. If you are using enough trimethoprim that certainly is the case.

Kunin That I agree with, but if one is using turbidimetric measures which are not reflecting antibacterial activity then I am confused.

Greenwood No, with sulphonamides and trimethoprim and also with nalidixic acid, the increase in opacity precedes bacterial death. But again, in the bladder model this is not a problem. Since the model is a dilution system, once the bacteria stop growing they are washed away and the opacity declines.

Mawer I would like to refer to synergy between penicillins and aminoglycosides. In the patient we may not have control over the relative concentration ratios at any particular time, but we control the time of administration. Is there any purpose in delaying the administration of an aminoglycoside in bacterial endocarditis until a certain period after the administration of the penicillin, or should the two be administered simultaneously?

Greenwood The effect of the penicillin is clearly to let the aminoglycoside in. However, there is evidence that when enterococci are exposed sequentially to penicillin, then streptomycin, you don't get synergy. In a recent study we confirmed this for penicillin and gentamicin and showed that the two antibiotics must be simultaneously present if "persisters" (bacteria surviving prolonged exposure to penicillins) are to be killed. If "persisters" are a cause of treatment failure, then in-vitro studies suggest that penicillin and aminoglycoside must be present together to dispose of this fraction of the population.

Jackson There are two theoretical bases for Professor Mawer's question which need to be separated. One is that the first drug, given ahead of time, might, in some circumstances, antagonize bacterial killing. For example, if you put tetracycline in first then you may negate the effect of penicillin, whereas if you do it the other way round an enhanced effect may be obtained. The second point concerns inoculum size. The use of one drug may reduce the inoculum size remarkably and the effect of the second drug might become appreciably altered. However, there is no evidence of which I am aware that either of these circumstances, *in vitro* or *in vivo*, are applicable to penicillin and aminoglycoside activity.

It has been said several times that the effect of penicillin on aminoglycosides is to accelerate the penetration of the aminoglycoside into the cell. I think it is naive to view bacteria in terms of making the cell wall or membrane leaky and then, by simple passive diffusion, aminoglycosides have access to the inside. This is a concept that doesn't have any biological substance because aminoglycosides utilize an energy-requiring process to put them inside the cell. Unless someone generates evidence to the effect that aminoglycosides are concentrated more easily or more rapidly in the presence of penicillin, the penetration idea is unfounded. From the studies that have been done, that I am familiar with, the answer is negative.

Greenwood So what, then, is the mechanism of synergy?

Jackson There are two or three possibilities. One of them is that aminoglycosides secure the reduced inoculum achieved by penicillin. If you decrease your population using penicillin and the antibiotic concentration then falls regrowth would occur under ordinary circumstances. The aminoglycoside can prevent that regrowth.

Another possible mechanism is that antibiotics do have some kind of additive function at the same cell independent of one making it leaky or not.

Kunin I don't believe myself naive, Dr Jackson. I'd like your discussion in this regard of the experiments by Moellering and Weinberg (1971).

This is the first time I have heard a major criticism of their experiments. As I recall, they used radio-labelled drugs. They showed more uptake of the radio-labelled streptomycin by the cells in the presence of penicillin. They were using gram-positive organisms *(Str. faecalis)*.

Brown I certainly think that Dr Greenwood's model which studies a culture which is being constantly diluted is an improvement on previous methods; but there are two aspects that might be defective from the point of view of the real in-vivo situation.

To what extent does the production of slime and the formation of micro-colonies in little pockets in the body contribute to the resistance of the cells? Simply being sequestered in a corner covered with slime might protect them from antibiotic action.

Secondly, there is the physiological state of bacteria growing in urine. If you have high populations, it could well be that one out of six or seven essential nutrients have run out and you are actually dealing with a nutrient-depleted culture. I would like to know if that is the case, and which nutrient it is, because the cells would be totally different depending on which nutrient it was.

My third point is that the envelope is very much an integrated structure, particularly with a gram-negative bacterium. The outer membrane, the peptidoglycan and the cytoplasmic membrane have very close relationships and disturbance of one portion disturbs the lot. Although aminoglycosides are taken up by the cytoplasmic membrane by a method requiring energy, they have got to get through the rest of the envelope before they reach the cytoplasmic membrane. Alteration of the peptidoglycan could disturb the outer membrane and aid penetration of the aminoglycosides.

Acar When you define synergism, there are a lot of observable antibacterial effects. Which effect should be measured to define the phenomenon—bacteriostasis, time to recovery, bactericidal effect? Is it possible to define a synergistic effect on the basis of one observable effect in antibacterial testing, or of more than one? Furthermore, it is difficult to get proof of a relationship between an effect observed *in vitro* and the clinical result.

Greenwood I want to get away from a discussion in which we try to tie synergy down to a particular definition. We have to look at each antibiotic combination in isolation and ask the question: "What is happening when these two antibiotics are together? In what way are they interacting?" and try and decide whether that is going to be clinically meaningful. Most interactions are discovered by accident, but having discovered the phenomenon a number of experimental observations can be brought to bear on the question of clinical relevance.

Acar I think it is important, in an in-vitro test, to know if the drugs are acting on one another or if the synergy is just one way. In sulphonamide–trimethoprim the sulphonamide acts on trimethoprim and trimethoprim acts on sulphonamide because in the chequerboard one has an effect on both sides. Between penicillin and streptomycin the effect is unidirectional, penicillin making streptomycin more bactericidal.

The minimum antibacterial concentration MAC puzzled me because it is a partial in-vitro effect. Should we use a percentage of the MIC rather than MAC. In bacteriology we are always going from maximum to minimum, which suggests a 100% effect which, as you know, is always so difficult to reach in experimental study.

Greenwood By MAC I mean the lowest concentration which causes a deviation from normal growth in the turbidimetric system; it is therefore a partial effect. I was using the MAC concept in two ways: (a) to point out that, as chessboard titrations employ sub-MIC concentrations, it is helpful to understand the nature of sub-MIC effects; (b) to try to estimate whether true biochemical synergy was occurring.

REFERENCE

Moellering, R. C. and Weinberg, A. N. (1971). Studies on antibiotic synergism against enterococci. II. Effect of various antibiotics on the uptake of ^{14}C-labelled streptomycin by enterococci. *Journal of Clinical Investigation* **50,** 2580.

Influence of the Bacterial Cell Envelope on Combined Antibiotic Action

MICHAEL R. W. BROWN

Department of Pharmacy,
University of Aston in Birmingham, Birmingham, UK.

PETER GILBERT

Department of Pharmacy,
University of Manchester, Manchester, UK.

and

RUTH M. M. KLEMPERER

Department of Pharmacy,
University of Aston in Birmingham, Birmingham, UK.

INTRODUCTION

Since the advent of chemotherapy, research has often been directed towards synergistic combinations of antimicrobial agents. Such combinations are vital for infections which fail to respond to single therapeutic agents and, in addition, may prevent the emergence of resistant mutants.

Several different rationales appear to underlie synergistic effects:

(i) drugs such as sulphamethoxazole and trimethoprim which act independently at different *loci* within a single pathway;
(ii) an enzyme inhibitor such as β-clavulanic acid which prevents a bacterial enzyme inactivating the effective drug;
(iii) a drug, which by interacting with the microbial cell envelope, allows increased penetration of a second drug to its target site.

To be effective, antimicrobial agents must be capable of achieving effective concentrations at their biochemical sites of action. Direct action upon the outermost surface of bacteria is rare; more commonly, lesions within the cell envelope or cell itself are implicated. Antibacterial agents must therefore be able to interact with and penetrate the cell envelope in order to exert their inhibitory action. Even drugs whose main site of action is cytoplasmic may also interact with and possibly change the envelope.

Studies of the properties of cell envelopes may explain the observed variation in drug sensitivities of different bacterial species to drug combinations, as for individual drugs. For example, the ratio of sulphamethoxazole to trimethoprim in cotrimoxazole is optimal for many species, but a quite different ratio is required for the genus *Neisseria* in parallel with different MICs (Bushby, 1969).

It is often difficult to predict with certainty the action of a drug combination in a particular case and in-vitro tests may not give results directly applicable to the in-vivo situation (Simmons, 1975). Recently there have been many developments regarding the important role of the bacterial envelope in resistance to drugs (Costerton and Cheng, 1975). In particular, it has been established that the bacterial envelope is remarkably plastic. When faced with the lack of an essential nutrient a dividing bacterium will manufacture an envelope characteristic of the particular depletion. The effect of different nutrient depletions, in addition to effects on general biochemistry, is to give rise to cells with radically different envelopes (Ellwood and Tempest, 1972; Holme, 1972). This phenomenon is particularly evident with respect to the outer membrane of gram-negative bacteria (Brown, 1975; Brown and Melling, 1969a,b).

Another potentially significant variable is that of growth rate. Bacterial doubling times during an infection may be slow and of the order of 20–24 h (Eudy and Burroughs, 1973; Meynell and Subbiah, 1963), rather than the 0·5–1.0 h more commonly obtained using complex laboratory media. For example, significant effects of growth rate and specific nutrient limitations on the sensitivity of *Pseudomonas aeruginosa* to drugs (Finch and Brown, 1975) have been demonstrated.

Any chemical or physiological stress that alters the cell envelope may enhance penetration of drugs and affect synergism, particularly where cell wall change by one of the drugs is important. It is this aspect of synergy that we wish to consider.

MODULATION OF DRUG EFFECTIVENESS BY THE CELL ENVELOPE

Bacterial cells differ from their mammalian counterparts in that they must interact with an ever-changing and often hostile environment. The effects of such adverse conditions may be compensated by changes in the cell envelope, i.e. cytoplasmic membrane, wall and, if present, slime layer (Fig. 1: simple diagram of gram-negative cell envelope).

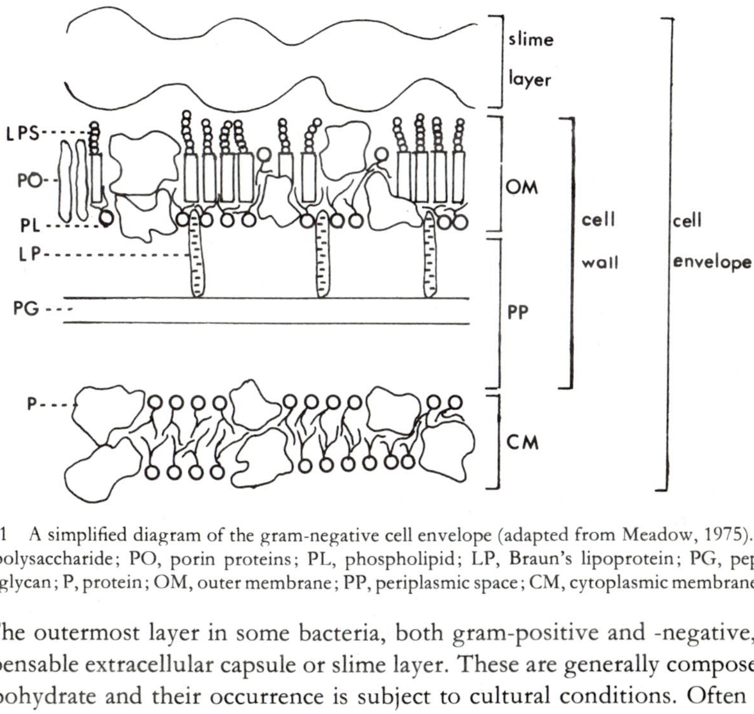

Fig. 1 A simplified diagram of the gram-negative cell envelope (adapted from Meadow, 1975). LPS, lipopolysaccharide; PO, porin proteins; PL, phospholipid; LP, Braun's lipoprotein; PG, peptidoglycan; P, protein; OM, outer membrane; PP, periplasmic space; CM, cytoplasmic membrane.

The outermost layer in some bacteria, both gram-positive and -negative, is a dispensable extracellular capsule or slime layer. These are generally composed of carbohydrate and their occurrence is subject to cultural conditions. Often they may occur as a diffuse slime surrounding and containing a number of microbial cells. The physiological role of such materials remains unclear, but they must confer advantages upon cells with respect to adhesion, colonization of surfaces, microcolony formation and resistance to phagocytosis (Costerton *et al.*, 1978). In addition they may represent a considerable barrier to drug penetration. Indeed, mucoid variants of *Ps. aeruginosa* may be selectively cultured by utilizing their enhanced resistance to penicillins (Govan, 1976). Clearly a drug which inhibits the polymerases associated with capsule/slime production is likely to be synergistic with a variety of antibiotics. Furthermore, such an action would influence adhesion, which is important in the initial stages of infection.

The cell wall is an integral part of the cell, which modulates the entry of antimicrobial agents in much the same way as it affects access of nutrients to the underlying cytoplasmic membrane. There are two distinct mechanisms involved in such action. The cytoplasmic membrane is bathed in a hydrophilic medium which is continuous with that of the extracellular environment. The peptidoglycan matrix in gram-positive bacteria (Scherrer and Gerhardt, 1971) and in conjunction with the outer membrane in gram-negatives (Nikaido, 1976; Nikaido and Nakae, 1979) functions as a molecular sieve, reducing the free diffusion of large hydrophilic molecules to the underlying cytoplasmic membrane. When direct access to the cytoplasmic membrane is denied, a drug must interact directly with the cell wall in order to traverse it. With gram-negative bacteria this may involve sequential partitioning across the lipophilic layers that constitute the outer membrane. A consideration of the structure of the bacterial wall must therefore form a basis for considering combined drug action.

The Passage of Antibiotics Through the Gram-positive Cell Wall

The gram-positive cell wall is composed of a complex, cross-linked network of peptidoglycan incorporating teichoic and teichuronic acids (Gerhardt and Judge, 1964; Hess and Lagg, 1958). Its function as a molecular sieve for large hydrophilic molecules depends upon the thickness of the matrix and the degree of cross-linking (Mitchell, 1959; Scherrer and Gerhardt, 1971). Both of these properties are variable and depend upon the growth rate and physiological status of the cells (Soloman, 1968). Due to its unique status as a bacterial polymer, peptidoglycan provides a major target for selective drug action. Indeed, many antibiotics act either directly upon it or interfere with its biosynthesis. Sub-lethal concentrations of such agents greatly perturb peptidoglycan structure. Decreases in the degree of cross-linking, such as might be associated with penicillin action at low concentration (Tipper and Strominger, 1965) must inevitably increase the porosity of the cell wall and enhance penetration of larger hydrophilic molecules to the cytoplasmic membrane. The well-known synergism of penicillin and streptomycin has been shown to be associated with an increased uptake of streptomycin in *Escherichia coli* (Plotz and Davis, 1962) and Moellering *et al.* (1971) found that a variety of drugs which inhibit stages in cell wall synthesis—cycloserine, vancomycin, bacitracin and cephalothin—as well as penicillin, were synergistic with streptomycin against enterococci.

The peptidoglycan is able to exclude only large polymeric materials (100 000 daltons) (Scherrer and Gerhardt, 1971) and fortunately most antimicrobials fall beneath this size limitation. Molecular sieving is, however, enhanced by the presence of charged groups within the peptidoglycan complex (Marquis, 1968). This, and the large surface area afforded by the cell wall, allows it to function like an ion-exchange column, strongly charged drug molecules being actively removed from solution as they diffuse through the matrix. Incoming molecules, including antibiotics, would have to saturate all unoccupied binding sites on the peptidoglycan surface before reaching the cytoplasmic membrane, just as gentamicin must saturate all the many binding sites on the polysaccharide fibres before it can pass through a cellulose filter (Wagman *et al.*, 1975). Subtle changes in the composition of the cell wall might markedly alter such adsorption phenomenon. For example, magnesium-limitation has been shown to cause increased affinity of *Bacillus subtilis* cell walls for Mg^{2+} adsorption. These changes correlated with alteration in wall teichoic and teichuronic acid content (Meers and Tempest, 1970). Similarly Tempest *et al.* (1968) showed that phosphate-limited and magnesium-limited *B. subtilis* had walls that were chemically substantially different. It is probable that such changes would markedly affect the ability of drugs to penetrate to the cytoplasmic membrane. Little work has been done in this area; therefore the practical significance of such effects is unknown. However, exclusion mechanisms of resistance have been implicated in gram-positive cells towards some preservatives (Gilbert and Brown, 1979; Hamilton, 1970).

The Passage of Antibiotics Through the Gram-negative Cell Wall

Permeation of the gram-negative cell wall by drugs is much more complex. The structure of the gram-negative outer membrane (OM) is now understood in molecular detail, not least through the excellent work of Nikaido and colleagues (Nikaido, 1976; Nikaido *et al.*, 1977). It has been the subject of several comprehensive reviews (Costerton, 1977; Nikaido and Nakae, 1979). The cell wall (Fig. 2) consists typically of an asymmetric lipid membrane bilayer attached via Braun's lipoproteins and possibly porin proteins to a thin matrix of peptidoglycan (Nikaido and Nakae, 1979). The exterior surface of the lipid bilayer is composed largely of closely packed lipopolysaccharide (LPS), orientated so that the hydrophilic polysaccharide portion is exposed to the surrounding medium and envelopes the cell surface. The lipophilic regions are directed inwards and interact with the fatty-acid chains of a phospholipid monolayer constituting the inner surface of the OM. Stability of the OM/peptidoglycan complex is maintained by divalent cation bridges (De Pamphilis, 1971; Schnaitman, 1971a,b) and lipoprotein (Costerton *et al.*, 1974). In *Ps. aeruginosa* there is some evidence that Braun's lipoprotein is much reduced or even absent (Meadow, 1975). Presumably divalent cation bridges play a relatively more important stabilizing role in this organism. Hence the potential of ion-chelators such as EDTA in combined therapy. Whilst combinations of EDTA and antibiotics are probably not suitable for systemic use, in-vitro studies (Weiser *et al.*, 1968; Weiser *et al.*, 1969) indicate their potential for the treatment of topical infections, particularly with *Ps. aeruginosa*. Some success has been reported *in vivo* (Goldschmidt *et al.*, 1972; Wooley *et al.*, 1974).

Wild-type strains of *E. coli, Salmonella typhimurium* and related gram-negative

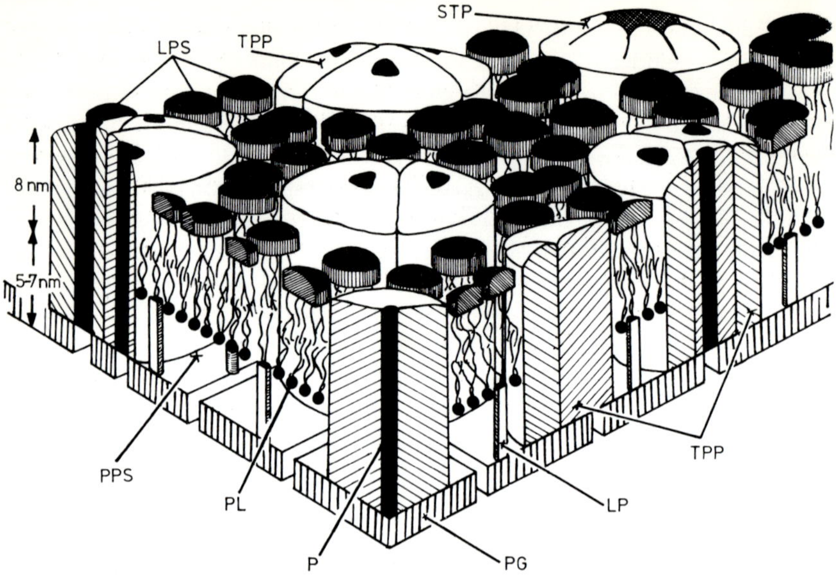

Fig. 2 A tentative structure of the gram-negative cell wall (adapted from Nikaido and Nakae, 1979). LPS, lipopolysaccharide (the oligosaccharide chains extending from the LPS into the external environment are omitted for visual clarity); TPP, trimer of porin protein; STP, specific transport protein; PPS, periplasmic space; PL, phospholipid; P, hydrophilic pore; PG, peptidoglycan; LP, Braun's lipoprotein.

organisms are characteristically sensitive to a number of antibiotics including neomycin, cycloserine, ampicillin and cephalothin. Alteration of LPS polysaccharide chain length does not affect sensitivity to these agents, but does alter sensitivity to a number of more hydrophobic agents, such as novobiocin, rifamycin and erythromycin (Leive, 1974; Roantree *et al.*, 1977; Tamaki *et al.*, 1971). Since the OM is the only part of the cell containing LPS in significant quantities, and the target for these agents is the cytoplasmic membrane or cytoplasm, the data suggests that at least two diffusion pathways function across the OM: one for hydrophobic drugs affected by LPS structure and at least one other for hydrophilic molecules (Nikaido, 1976; Nikaido and Nakae, 1979).

Hydrophilic drugs

Together the phospholipid and LPS form a classical lipid bilayer and constitute a formidable barrier to the penetration of hydrophilic molecules, nutrients and hydrophilic drugs alike. Hydrophilic nutrients, however, traverse the cell envelope by two distinct mechanisms, mediated in both cases by the presence of outer-membrane proteins. The transport of some materials may be facilitated by specific transport proteins located across the outer membrane. Such carrier proteins are analogous to those of the cytoplasmic membrane and are highly specific in their action (Hantke, 1976; Hancock *et al.*, 1976; Sabet and Schnaitman, 1973; Wookey and Rosenberg, 1978) and might be involved in the transport of small molecules such as iron (Pugsley and Reeves, 1976; Wayne *et al.*, 1976). Less specific is the action of the porin proteins (Decad and Nikaido, 1976; Nakae and Nikaido, 1975; Payne and Gilvarg, 1968). Evidence suggests that these porin proteins are aggregated (Palva and Randall, 1978) within the outer membrane as trimers, and that each trimer forms a hydrophilic water-filled pore allowing the passive diffusion of small hydrophilic molecules (Nikaido and Nakae, 1979). Specificity and rate of transpore diffusion depends upon molecular size (Nikaido and Nakae, 1979), charge (Stock *et al.*, 1977) and, for molecules approaching the maximum size limit, lipophilicity (Nikaido, 1976; Nikaido and Nakae, 1979; Zimmerman and Rosselet, 1977). On the basis of transpore diffusion rates Nikaido (1976) suggested that the diameter of these pores was approximately 1.2 nm.

Hydrophobic drugs

Most biological membranes allow transmembrane diffusion of small hydrophobic molecules (Danielli, 1952). The OM of many wild type gram-negative bacteria is probably exceptional in that hydrophobic compounds are excluded partly by the surface hydrophilic polysaccharides and partly by the close stacking of the LPS which hinders access to the hydrophobic centre of the OM. This stacking is aided by the relative lack of phospholipid (Nikaido and Nakae, 1979). The OMs of deep rough gram-negative microorganisms resemble typical biological membranes more closely. Hydrophobic compounds are able to traverse the layered structure of the OM through the combined action of oil/water partitioning and passive diffusion processes (Stein, 1967). Hansch (1973), Hansch and Fujita (1964), and Lien *et al.* (1968) argued that the differences in biological activity of chemically related antimicrobials, acting at similar sites within the cell, would be a reflection of their relative ease of penetration through the various lipid barriers of the cells and their ability to react when at that site. The outer components of the cell were considered as a series of aqueous and lipophilic layers. Substances of low water solubility would be unable to penetrate these aqueous layers, and could accumulate within the lipid region (Parker and McRobbie, 1974); similarly those with low oil solubility would be unable to cross the lipophilic barriers. Compounds between these two extremes must exist which possess the optimum balance between hydrophilicity and lipophilicity for traversing the cell's barriers. Therefore if log P (log oil/water partition coefficient) were plotted against the biological activity of a series of compounds then a parabolic relationship ought to be obtained, log P_0 being the value of log P for the compound with optimal activity. Many such parabolic relationships have been demonstrated (Hansch and Fujita, 1964). In this fashion it is possible to determine the optimal lipophilicity of a drug for outer membrane permeation. The overall value of log P_0 for a congeneric series of drugs was found to be approximately 4·0 for gram-negative microorganisms and 6·0 for gram-positives (Lien *et al.*, 1968). This difference was attributed to the gram-negative wall.

The idea of optimal drug lipophilicity can be related to drug combinations passing through the cell envelope. Perturbation of LPS by one agent (e.g. EDTA) may markedly increase the activity of another (Leive, 1974). Figure 3 represents a compartmental model for drug disposition in the gram-negative cell. If one drug disturbs one rate process within a series of hydrophilic/lipophilic compartments then log P_0 for the activity of another drug may vary (Hansch, 1973). Drugs are rarely selected on the basis of optimal activity alone, rather on a balance between the toxicity and activity. Small changes in log P_0 might markedly increase drug activity without necessarily increasing toxicity to the patient.

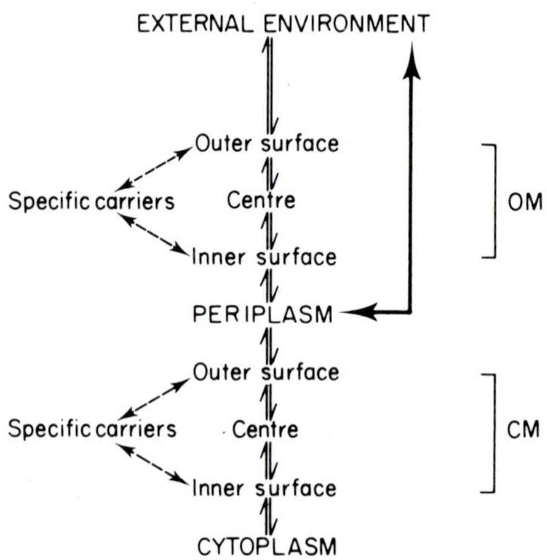

Fig. 3 A compartmental model describing drug disposition in a gram-negative bacterium. OM, outer membrane; CM, cytoplasmic membrane; ←---→ transport by specific carrier proteins; ⇌, diffusion and partitioning; ←→ diffusion through hydrophilic pores.

VARIATION IN DRUG SENSITIVITY WITH VARIATION IN THE CELL ENVELOPE

The bacterial cell envelope is remarkably flexible both in structure and in composition. Changes in envelope phospholipid (Benns and Proulx, 1974; Günter *et al.*, 1975), LPS (Dean *et al.*, 1977); Tempest and Ellwood, 1969), protein (Ames *et al.*, 1974; Koplow and Goldfine, 1974), fatty acid (Minnikin *et al.*, 1971a,b) and cation content (Kenward *et al.*, 1978) often accompany the effects of nutrient depletion and/or growth rate; all may confer survival advantage on the cells. Such effects markedly influence drug sensitivity by affecting the permeability properties of the envelope (Brown, 1975; Brown and Melling, 1969a,b, 1975; Gilbert and Brown, 1978a,b).

Where drugs are synergistic by acting at different *loci* in the same pathway, then a change in the permeation of either is likely to modify their synergistic action only to the extent that it affects individual drug action. However, where one drug modifies the cell wall allowing increased penetration by a second, then a change in the cell wall which affects the activity of the first drug may be expected to have a profound effect on its synergistic action with the second. Research in this area is still in its infancy and one can only predict possible effects on synergism from effects on individual drugs. For example, as the growth rate of carbon-limited *Ps. aeruginosa* is increased, it becomes more sensitive to EDTA or gentamicin, but shows no change in sensitivity to carbenicillin (Dean *et al.*, 1977). One might predict that the effectiveness of EDTA in combined therapy (Goldschmidt *et al.*, 1972; Wooley *et al.*, 1974) would vary with the growth rate of the infecting organisms. Indeed, some animal trials of EDTA with ampicillin or tetracycline as topical treatments for *Ps. aeruginosa* infections have proved disappointing (Weiser, 1973), although these combinations were effective in in-vitro tests and it was clear that lack of activity in the animal was not due to quenching of the EDTA by divalent ions. Carbenicillin and gentamicin are synergistic against *Ps. aeruginosa* (Sonne and Jawetz, 1969). Carbenicillin may potentiate gentamicin action (Plotz and Davis, 1962); if so, the effects of growth rate on the combination are unlikely to be greater than that attributable to the change in sensitivity to gentamicin.

Many of the environmentally induced changes which take place in the gram-negative envelope are in the OM and it is therefore not surprising that they markedly affect sensitivity of organisms to polymyxin (Brown and Melling, 1969b; Finch and Brown, 1975), a drug which interacts initially with the OM (Rosenthal and Storm, 1977) and is synergistic with a variety of antibiotics (Storm *et al.*, 1977). The use of the synergistic combination sulphamethoxazole–trimethoprim–polymyxin has been suggested for serious gram-negative infections (Rosenblatt and Stewart, 1974), and although some doubt has been cast on how much each drug increases the transport of the other in such mixtures (Handley *et al.*, 1974), it seems likely that phenotypic variations in the cell wall may have a big effect on the outcome of therapy. Chlorhexidine is another antibacterial agent synergistic with sulphonamides and combined topical use of chlorhexidine and sulphadiazine has been suggested for therapy of infected burns (Quesnel *et al.*, 1978). Chlorhexidine is also a membrane-active agent acting on the cell envelope, and the sensitivity of gram-negatives to it is similarly altered by nutrient depletion (Ismail *et al.*, 1977; Klemperer *et al.*, 1977).

The normal body defences are frequently an important component of successful therapy, but the environmental conditions which change the cell envelope and drug penetration may also affect the susceptibility of bacteria to these mechanisms. The susceptibility of *Ps. aeruginosa* to phagocytosis varies both with growth rate and with nutrient limitations (Finch and Brown, 1978). The importance of LPS in protecting smooth gram-negatives from the bactericidal activity of complement (Reynolds and Pruul, 1971) suggests that fluctuations in lipopolysaccharide (LPS) content resulting from changes in growth rate (Gilbert and Brown, 1978a) may affect the sensitivity of cells to it. Furthermore, complement and polymyxin are synergistic (Pruul and Reynolds, 1972), so that any reduction in sensitivity to either will be magnified. However, the OM does not appear to be a barrier to the more hydrophilic drugs tetracycline and streptomycin, and complement is not synergistic with these (Tseng and Bryan, 1974).

The nutritional status of microorganisms *in vivo* is difficult to assess (Brown, 1977). One may speculate about the nature of the growth-limiting nutrient of bacteria in various localized sites but little empirical information is available. Ellwood and Hunter (1977) have discussed the resemblance between the mouth and a chemostat for oral bacteria. Little is known about growth limitation in urine, although Anderson (1976) has pointed out the critical difference of urine pH, osmolality and constituents from laboratory media which can influence the physiological state of the bacteria and drug resistance. Broughton *et al.* (1968) reported on the fall in serum magnesium in a proportion of patients with burns. The magnesium concentration in the burns tissue was not reported but the practice of saline baths would probably have even further reduced magnesium levels in the burn and possibly influenced growth of bacteria. The reasons for the appearance and persistence of mucoid forms of *Ps. aeruginosa* in the lungs of cystic fibrosis patients (Doggett, 1969) are interesting. Environmental factors must be critical since they are rarely isolated from patients and usually revert to non-mucoid forms *in vitro* (Govan, 1975, 1976).

There is evidence that iron is normally growth-limiting in serum (Bullen *et al.*, 1974; Weinberg, 1978) and that infection may elicit the response of a drop in the concentration of iron available to invading organisms (Sussman, 1974). A similar in-vivo growth-limiting possibility has been suggested for inorganic phosphate or even zinc (Weinberg, 1974). There is little published work on the effects of iron limitation on bacterial structure and resistance (Light and Clegg, 1974). Nevertheless, slow-growing, iron-limited chemostat cultures may prove more relevant for testing drug combinations than the "overnight" broth cultures commonly used, which bear little relation to the in-vivo environment.

REFERENCES

Ames, F. L., Spudich, E. N. and Nikaido, H. (1974). Protein composition of the outer membrane of *Salmonella typhimurium*: Effect of lipopolysaccharide mutations. *Journal of Bacteriology* **117,** 406–416.

Anderson, J. D. (1976). The relevance of urine and serum antibacterial activity to the treatment of urinary tract infections. *Journal of Antimicrobial Chemotherapy* **2,** 226–228.
Benns, G. and Proulx, P. (1974). The effect of ATP and Mg^{2+} on the synthesis of phosphatidylglycerol in *Escherichia coli* preparations. *Biochimica et Biophysica Acta* **337,** 318–324.
Broughton, A., Anderson, I. R. M. and Bowden, C. H. (1968). Magnesium-deficiency syndrome in burns. *Lancet* **ii,** 1156–1158.
Brown, M. R. W. (1975). The role of the envelope in resistance. *In* "Resistance of *Pseudomonas aeruginosa,*" 71–107. (Ed. M. R. W. Brown), Wiley, London.
Brown, M. R. W. (1977). Nutrient depletion and antibiotic susceptibility. *Journal of Antimicrobial Chemotherapy* **3,** 198–201.
Brown, M. R. W. and Melling, J. (1969a). Loss of sensitivity to EDTA by *Pseudomonas aeruginosa* grown under conditions of magnesium-limitation. *Journal of General Microbiology* **54,** 439–444.
Brown, M. R. W. and Melling, J. (1969b). Role of divalent cations in the action of polymyxin B and EDTA on *Pseudomonas aeruginosa. Journal of General Microbiology* **59,** 263–274.
Brown, M. R. W. and Melling, J. (1975). The effect of the bacterial environment upon resistance. *In* "Resistance of *Pseudomonas aeruginosa,*" 35–70. (Ed. M. R. W. Brown), Wiley, London.
Bullen, J. J., Rogers, H. J. and Griffiths, E. (1974). Bacterial iron metabolism in infection and immunity. *In* "Microbial Iron Metabolism: A Comprehensive Treatise," 517. (Ed. J. B. Neilands), Academic Press, London and New York.
Bushby, S. R. M. (1969). Combined antibacterial action *in vitro* of trimethoprim and sulphonamides. The *in vitro* nature of synergy. *Postgraduate Medical Journal* **45** (Supplt), 10–18.
Costerton, J. W. (1977). Cell envelope as a barrier to antibiotics. *In* "Microbiology," 151–157. American Society for Microbiology, Washington D.C.
Costerton, J. W. and Cheng, K.-J. (1975). The role of the bacterial envelope in antibiotic resistance. *Journal of Antimicrobial Chemotherapy* **1,** 363–377.
Costerton, J. W., Geesey, G. G. and Cheng, K.-J. (1978). How bacteria stick. *Scientific American* **238,** 86–95.
Costerton, J. W., Ingram, J. M. and Cheng, K.-J. (1974). Structure and function of the cell envelope of gram-negative bacteria. *Bacteriological Reviews* **38,** 87–110.
Danielli, J. F. (1952). *In* "The Permeability of Natural Membranes," 80–104. (Eds. H. Dawson and J. F. Danielli), Cambridge University Press. London.
Dean, A. C. R., Ellwood, D. C., Melling, J. and Robinson, A. (1977). The action of antibacterial agents on bacteria grown in continuous culture. *In* "Continuous Culture 6: Applications and New Fields," 251–261 (Eds. A. C. R. Dean, D. C. Ellwood, C. G. T. Evans and J. Melling), Ellis Horwood, Chichester.
Decad, G. and Nikaido, H. (1976). Outer-membrane of gram-negative bacteria. XII. Molecular-sieving function of cell wall. *Journal of Bacteriology* **128,** 325–336.
De Pamphilis, M. C. (1971). Dissociation and reassembly of *Escherichia coli* outer membrane and of lipopolysaccharide and their reassembly on to flagellar basal bodies. *Journal of Bacteriology* **105,** 1184–1199.
Doggett, R. G. (1969). Incidence of mucoid *Pseudomonas aeruginosa* from clinical sources. *Applied Microbiology* **18,** 936–937.
Ellwood, D. C. and Hunter, J. R. (1977). The mouth as a chemostat. *In* "Continuous Culture 6: Applications and New Fields," 270–282 (Eds. A. C. R. Dean, D. C. Ellwood, C. G. T. Evans and J. Melling), Ellis Horwood, Chichester, England.
Ellwood, D. C. and Tempest, D. W. (1972). Effects of environment on bacterial wall content and composition. *Advances in Microbial Physiology* **7,** 83–117.
Eudy, W. W. and Burroughs, S. E. (1973). Generation times of *Proteus mirabilis* and

Escherichia coli in experimental infections. *Chemotherapy* **19,** 161–170.

Finch, J. E. and Brown, M. R. W. (1975). The influence of nutrient-limitation in a chemostat on the sensitivity of *Pseudomonas aeruginosa* to polymyxin and EDTA. *Journal of Antimicrobial Chemotherapy* **1,** 379–386.

Finch, J. E. and Brown, M. R. W. (1978). Effect of growth environment on *Pseudomonas aeruginosa* killing by rabbit polymorphonuclear leukocytes and cationic proteins. *Infection and Immunity* **20,** 340–346.

Gerhardt, P. and Judge, J. A. (1964). Porosity of isolated cell walls of *Saccharomyces cerevisiae* and *Bacillus megaterium*. *Journal of Bacteriology* **87,** 945–995.

Gilbert, P. and Brown, M. R. W. (1978a). Influence of growth rate and nutrient limitation on the gross cellular composition of *Pseudomonas aeruginosa* and its resistance to 3- and 4-chlorophenol. *Journal of Bacteriology* **133,** 1066–1072.

Gilbert, P. and Brown, M. R. W. (1978b). Effect of R-plasmid RP1 and nutrient depletion on the gross cellular composition of *Escherichia coli* and its resistance to some uncoupling phenols. *Journal of Bacteriology* **133,** 1062–1065.

Gilbert, P. and Brown, M. R. W. (1979). Changes in drug sensitivity of *Bacillus megaterium* associated with growth rate and nutrient limitation. *Society for General Microbiology Quarterly* **6,** 94.

Goldschmidt, M. C., Kuhn, C. R., Perry, K. and Johnson, D. E. (1972). EDTA and lysozyme lavage in the treatment of *Pseudomonas* and bladder infections. *Journal of Urology* **107,** 969–972.

Govan, J. R. W. (1975). Mucoid strains of *Pseudomonas aeruginosa*: the influence of culture medium on the stability of mucus production. *Journal of Medical Microbiology* **8,** 513–522.

Govan, J. R. W. (1976). Antibiotic therapy and cystic fibrosis: increased resistance of mucoid *Pseudomonas aeruginosa* to carbenicillin. *Journal of Antimicrobial Chemotherapy* **2,** 215–217.

Günter, T., Richter, L. and Schmalbeck, J. (1975). Phospholipids of *Escherichia coli* in magnesium deficiency. *Journal of General Microbiology* **86,** 191–193.

Hamilton, W. A. (1970). The mode of action of membrane active antibacterials. *FEBS Symposium* **20,** 71–79.

Hancock, R. E. W., Hantke, K. and Braun, V. (1976). Iron transport in *Escherichia coli* K12: involvement of the colicin B receptor and of a citrate inducible protein. *Journal of Bacteriology* **127,** 1370–1375.

Handley, P. S., Quesnel, L. B. and Sturgiss, M. M. (1974). Ultrastructural changes produced in *Proteus vulgaris* by a synergistic combination of colistin and sulphadiazine. *Microbios* **10,** 211–223.

Hansch, C. (1973). Quantitative approaches to pharmacological structure–activity relationships. *In* "Structure–Activity Relationships," Vol I (Ed. C. J. Cavallito), Pergamon, Oxford.

Hansch, C. and Fujita, T. (1964). A method for the correlation of biological activity and chemical structure. *Journal of the American Chemical Society* **86,** 1616–1626.

Hantke, K. (1976). Phage T6—colicin K receptor and nucleoside transport in *Escherichia coli*. *FEBS Letters* **70,** 109–112.

Hess, E. L. and Lagg, S. E. (1958). Some physical aspects of the bacterial cell. *Science (N.Y.)* **128,** 356–358.

Holme, T. (1972). Influence of environment on the content and composition of bacterial envelopes. *Journal of Applied Chemistry and Biotechnology* **22,** 391–399.

Ismail, N. T. A. J., Klemperer, R. M. M. and Brown, M. R. W. (1977). Resistance of *Escherichia coli* to disinfectants: influence of R-plasmid RP1 and nutrient depletion. *Journal of Applied Bacteriology* **43,** xvi–xvii.

Kenward, M. A., Brown, M. R. W. and Fryer, J. J. (1978). The effect of divalent metal cations on composition and drug resistance of *Pseudomonas aeruginosa* NCTC 6750. *Abstracts of the Annual Meeting, American Society for Microbiology* A7.

Klemperer, R. M. M., Al-Dujaili, D. A., Lawson, J. J. and Brown, M. R. W. (1977). The effect of nutrient depletion on the resistance of *Proteus mirabilis* to antibacterial agents. *Journal of Applied Bacteriology* **43,** xvi.

Koplow, J. and Goldfine, H. (1974). Alterations in the outer membrane of the cell envelope of heptose-deficient mutants of *Escherichia coli*. *Journal of Bacteriology* **117,** 527–543.

Leive, L. (1974). The barrier function of the gram-negative envelope. *Annals of the New York Academy of Sciences* **235,** 109–129.

Lien, E. J., Hansch, C. and Anderson, S. M. (1968). Structure–activity correlations for antibacterial agents of gram-positive and gram-negative cells. *Journal of Medicinal Chemistry* **11,** 430–441.

Light, P. A. and Clegg, R. A. (1974). Metabolism in iron-limited growth. *In* "Microbial Iron Metabolism: a Comprehensive Treatise," 35. (Ed. J. B. Neilands), Academic Press, London and New York.

Marquis, R. E. (1968). Salt-induced contraction of bacterial cell walls. *Journal of Bacteriology* **95,** 775–781.

Meadow, P. M. (1975). Wall and membrane structures in the genus *Pseudomonas*. *In* "Genetics and Biochemistry of *Pseudomonas*" 67–98 (Eds. P. H. Clarke and M. H. Richmond), Wiley, Chichester.

Meers, J. L. and Tempest, D. W. (1970). The influence of growth-limiting substrate and medium NaCl concentration on the synthesis of magnesium-binding sites in the walls of *Bacillus subtilis* var *niger*. *Journal of General Microbiology* **63,** 325–331.

Meynell, G. G. and Subbiah, T. V. (1963). The true division and death rates of *Salmonella typhimurium* in the mouse spleen determined with superinfecting phage 22. *British Journal of Experimental Pathology* **44,** 197–219.

Minnikin, D. E., Abdulrahimzadeh, H. and Baddiley, J. (1971a). The interrelation of phosphatidylethanolamine and glycosyldiglycerides in bacterial membranes. *Biochemical Journal* **124,** 447–448.

Minnikin, D. E., Abdulrahimzadeh, H. and Baddiley, J. (1971b). The interrelation of polar lipids in bacterial membranes. *Biochimica et Biophysica Acta* **249,** 651–655.

Mitchell, P. (1959). Biochemical cytology of microorganisms. *Annual Review of Microbiology* **13,** 407–440.

Moellering, R. C., Wennersten, C. and Weinberg, A. N. (1971). Studies on antibiotic synergism against enterococci. 1. Bacteriologic studies. *Journal of Laboratory and Clinical Medicine* **77,** 821–827.

Nakae, T. and Nikaido, H. (1975). Outer membrane as a diffusion barrier in *Salmonella typhimurium*. *Journal of Biological Chemistry* **250,** 7359–7365.

Nikaido, H. (1976). Outer membrane of *Salmonella typhimurium*: transmembrane diffusion of some hydrophobic substances. *Biochimica et Biophysica Acta* **433,** 118–132.

Nikaido, H. and Nakae, T. (1979). The outer membrane of gram-negative bacteria. *Advances in Microbial Physiology*. In press.

Nikaido, H., Song, S. A., Shaltiel, L. and Nurimen, M. (1977). Outer membrane of *Salmonella* XIV. Reduced transmembrane diffusion rates in porin-deficient mutants. *Biochemical and Biophysical Research Communications* **76,** 324–330.

Palva, E. T. and Randall, L. L. (1978). Arrangement of protein I in *Escherichia coli* outer membrane: cross-linking study. *Journal of Bacteriology* **133,** 279–286.

Parker, M. S. and McRobbie, D. I. (1974). Some aspects of the antifungal activity of esters of *p*-hydroxybenzoic acid. *International Biodeterioration Bulletin* **10,** 109–113.

Payne, J. W. and Gilvarg, C. (1968). Size restriction on peptide utilization in *Escherichia coli*. *Journal of Biological Chemistry* **243,** 6291–6299.

Plotz, P. H. and Davis, B. D. (1962). Synergism between streptomycin and penicillin: A proposed mechanism. *Science (N.Y.)* **135,** 1067–1068.

Pruul, H. and Reynolds, B. L. (1972). Interaction of complement and polymyxin with gram-negative bacteria. *Infection and Immunity* **6,** 709–717.

Pugsley, A. P. and Reeves, P. (1976). Iron uptake in colicin-B-resistant mutants of *Escherichia coli* K-12. *Journal of Bacteriology* **126,** 1052–1062.

Quesnel, L. B., Al-Najjar, A. R. and Buddhavudhikrai, P. (1978). Synergism between chlorhexidine and sulphadiazine. *Journal of Applied Bacteriology* **45,** 397–405.

Reynolds, B. L. and Pruul, H. (1971). Protective role of smooth lipopolysaccharide in the serum bactericidal reaction. *Infection and Immunity* **4,** 764–771.

Roantree, R. J., Kuo, T.-T. and MacPhee, D. G. (1977). The effect of defined lipopolysaccharide core defects upon antibiotic resistances of *Salmonella typhimurium*. *Journal of General Microbiology* **103,** 223–234.

Rosenblatt, J. E. and Stewart, P. R. (1974). Combined activity of sulfamethoxazole, trimethoprim, and polymyxin B against gram-negative bacilli. *Antimicrobial Agents and Chemotherapy* **6,** 84–92.

Rosenthal, K. S. and Storm, D. R. (1977). Disruption of the *Escherichia coli* outer membrane permeability barrier by immobilized polymyxin B. *Journal of Antibiotics* **30,** 1087–1092.

Sabet, S. F. and Schnaitman, C. A. (1973). Purification and properties of the colicin E receptor of *Escherichia coli*. *Journal of Biological Chemistry* **248,** 1797–1806.

Scherrer, R. and Gerhardt, P. (1971). Molecular sieving by the *Bacillus megaterium* cell wall and protoplast. *Journal of Bacteriology* **107,** 718–735.

Schnaitman, C. A. (1971a). Solubilization of the cytoplasmic membrane of *Escherichia coli* by Triton X100. *Journal of Bacteriology* **108,** 545–552.

Schnaitman, C. A. (1971b). Effect of ethylenediaminetetraacetic acid, Triton X100 and lysozyme on the morphology and chemical composition of isolated walls of *Escherichia coli*. *Journal of Bacteriology* **108,** 533–563.

Simmons, N. A. (1975). Antibiotic synergy. *Journal of Antimicrobial Chemotherapy* **1,** 257–261.

Soloman, A. K. (1968). Characterisation of biological membranes by equivalent pores. *Journal of General Physiology* **51,** 335–354.

Sonne, M. and Jawetz, E. (1969). Combined action of carbenicillin and gentamicin on *Pseudomonas aeruginosa in vitro*. *Applied Microbiology* **17,** 893–896.

Stein, W. D. (1967). "The Movement of Molecules Across Cell Membranes." Academic Press, New York and London.

Stock, J. B., Rauch, B. and Roseman, S. (1977). Periplasmic space in *Salmonella typhimurium* and *Escherichia coli*. *Journal of Biological Chemistry* **252,** 7850–7861.

Storm, D. R., Rosenthal, K. S. and Swanson, P. E. (1977). Polymyxin and related peptide antibiotics. *Annual Reviews of Biochemistry* **46,** 723–763.

Sussman, M. (1974). Iron and infection. *In* "Iron in Biochemistry and Medicine," 649 (Eds. A. Jacobs and M. Worwood), Academic Press, London and New York.

Tamaki, S., Sato, T. and Matsuhashi, M. (1971). Role of lipopolysaccharides in antibiotic resistance and bacteriophage adsorption of *Escherichia coli* K-12. *Journal of Bacteriology* **105,** 968–975.

Tempest, D. W., Dicks, J. W. and Ellwood, D. C. (1968). Influence of growth conditions on the concentration of potassium in *Bacillus subtilis* var. *niger* and its possible relationship to cellular ribonucleic acid, teichoic acid and teichuronic acid. *Biochemical Journal* **106,** 237–243.

Tempest, D. W. and Ellwood, D. C. (1969). The influence of growth conditions on the composition of some cell wall components of *Aerobacter aerogenes. Biotechnology Bioengineering* **11,** 775–783.

Tipper, D. J. and Strominger, J. L. (1965). Mechanism of action of penicillins—proposal based on their structural similarity to acyl-D-alanyl-D-alanine. *Proceedings of the National Academy of Sciences, U.S.A.* **54,** 1133–1141.

Tseng, J. T. and Bryan, L. E. (1974). The effect of complement and other cell wall reagents on tetracycline and streptomycin resistance in *Pseudomonas aeruginosa. Canadian Journal of Microbiology* **20,** 1101–1107.

Wagman, G. H., Bailey, J. V. and Weinstein, M. J. (1975). Binding of aminoglycoside antibiotics to filtration materials. *Antimicrobial Agents and Chemotherapy* **7,** 316–319.

Wayne, R., Erick, K. and Neilands, J. B. (1976). Evidence for common binding sites for ferrichrome compounds and bacteriophage Φ80 in the cell envelope of *Escherichia coli. Journal of Bacteriology* **121,** 497–503.

Weinberg, E. D. (1974). Iron and susceptibility to infectious disease. *Science (N.Y.)* **184,** 952–956.

Weinberg, E. D. (1978). Iron and infection. *Microbiological Reviews* **42,** 45–66.

Weiser, R. (1973). Combinations of edetic acid and antibiotics in the treatment of rat burns infected with a resistant strain of *Pseudomonas aeruginosa. Journal of Infectious Diseases* **128,** 566–569.

Weiser, R., Asscher, A. W. and Wimpenny, J. (1968). In-vitro reversal of antibiotic resistance by ethylenediaminetetraacetic acid. *Nature (London)* **219,** 1365–1366.

Weiser, R., Wimpenny, J. and Asscher, A. W. (1969). Synergistic effect of edetic acid/antibiotic combinations on *Pseudomonas aeruginosa. Lancet* **ii,** 619–620.

Wookey, P. and Rosenberg, H. (1978). Involvement of inner and outer membrane components in the transport of iron and colicin B action in *Escherichia coli. Journal of Bacteriology* **133,** 661–666.

Wooley, R. E., Schall, W. D., Eagon, R. G. and Scott, T. A. (1974). The efficacy of EDTA-tris-lysozyme lavage in the treatment of experimentally induced *Pseudomonas aeruginosa* cystitis in the dog. *American Journal of Veterinary Medicine* **35,** 27–29.

Zimmerman, W. and Rosselet, A. (1977). Function of the outer membrane of *Escherichia coli* as a permeability barrier to beta-lactam antibiotics. *Antimicrobial Agents and Chemotherapy* **12,** 368–372.

DISCUSSION

O'Grady I was interested in Professor Brown's comments on slime and microcolony formation and would like to answer the question which he raised about the bladder model because one aspect we have been particularly interested in is the adhesion of organisms to the glass surface. They not only stick to grass in the streams, but they stick to glass in the vessels and no doubt to the chemostat as well. This has been a problem to us in that if we run the experiment for long periods we get growth on the opacity chamber and the opacity reading no longer reflects the changes in the broth. However, there are reasons for believing clinically from mathematical modelling and from the behaviour of the model that organisms growing on the surface contribute significantly to the persistence of infection. It is also possible that they respond quite differently to antimicrobial agents from those which are growing in the fluid culture.

Brown I agree. No one wishes to work on bacteria stuck on the surface of the culture vessel but if you could actually study them instead of regarding them as a nuisance, I am sure that would be more useful than anything.

Asscher Your work implies that if you make bacteria sick by limiting the food supply they become susceptible to antimicrobials. You asked whether nutrient limitation had been used in clinical practice. If one grows organisms in urine to the maximum population and removes the organisms by centrifugation, you can grow them in that same urine again. It follows that nutrient limitation as a means of controlling infection is likely to be very difficult. Some years ago we tried to reduce the amount of calcium in the urine to control *Pseudomonas* infection because this organism becomes exceedingly sensitive to a number of antibiotics if you deplete the medium of calcium and/or magnesium. We went so far as to infuse patients with *Pseudomonas* urinary tract infection with EDTA to see whether we could remove enough calcium from the urine. However, even when the patient developed tetany there was still enough urinary calcium for the *Pseudomonas* to remain resistant to penicillin G.

Then we decided to try calcium limitation on *Pseudomonas*-infected burns. Here we were successful in showing that *Pseudomonas* could be made very sensitive to ampicillin, but this could only be achieved on the surface of the burn and not in the deeper layers so that the animals, therefore, still died of *Pseudomonas* septicaemia.

We have done our best with nutrient limitation but it seems that human beings and microorganisms have too much in common in their nutrient requirements for the method to be effective.

Brown The vast majority of bacteria in the world must be limited by something. I don't understand the concept of "normal bacteria". I think it is normal to be "limited" or else to be growing exponentially.

Is there any site in the body where the environment is such that when a culture grows, it tends to run out of one component characteristically rather than another? In septicaemia it could be that iron depletion limits an organism's capacity to grow.

Your remarks about the urine are interesting but the bacteria could be oxygen limited; they could not have been running out of magnesium sulphate or nitrogen. But I just wonder whether at some other site in the body this is not the case.

In burned patients the magnesium level in the patient drops. But does it ever drop below the level that limits the growth of bacteria?

Kass One reasonable hypothesis is that the bacteria have stopped increasing in numbers because they have run out of nutrient; another is that certain metabolic products accumulate which inhibit multiplication. Which of these looks more likely in most situations? Accumulation of metabolic products seems to be a more likely explanation in most situations.

One can demonstrate that with an excess of glucose in the culture medium, the numbers of bacteria which grow nevertheless level off at pretty much the same point as they do with a much lower amount of glucose. Depletion only comes into play at certain points and the accumulation of metabolic products seems to be more constant here. This particularly applies in human tissues, where the amounts of most nutrients are in great excess. If one can see the phenomenon at work in urine, as Dr Asscher described, it will be even better in body tissues which are nutrient loaded.

Brown However, it is possible to grow populations densely with increased aeration so that the culture is like thick soup.

Kass I think this depends entirely on the system. With most acid-producing bacteria accumulation of metabolic acid accounts for the limitation of growth, so that neutralization alone is effective in stimulating multiplication for a few more cycles, until lack of substrate becomes limiting.

Brown We grow *E. coli* and have calibration curves for each of the essential nutrients. Incremental increases of glucose produce similar increments in the mass of cells produced. There are no more increases because in our system there is oxygen limitation. If we then increase aeration we can add more glucose and produce more cells. We have also done this with *Proteus*.

Kass I don't question its truth. I am simply saying that in most situations that is not the way it operates. It is the organic acid that causes growth to stop, usually before substrate has been exhausted. In part this depends upon the buffering capacity of the culture medium; and, of course, on the amount of acid produced and the relative resistance of individual bacteria to such acid.

Brown Perhaps the situations I am familiar with are not entirely typical.

Jackson I am not challenging the validity of the importance of nutrients but there must be additional controlling factors, most of which we probably don't know, but contact inhibition is one, i.e. control by the density of cells *per se*. A non-cancerous cell has very strong contact inhibition for some reasons that I don't think are clear. A non-cancerous cell growing in a medium that will permit its growth, suddenly at some number, will die. There is something in the genes of the cell that makes it stop at some time. It is not just simply nutrient, oxygen or pH change.

Kunin I would like to cite a more common example of the point you are making. Think of the manufacture of wine or beer. This is similar to a chemostat in that as the yeast multiplies it produces alcohol. Excess alcohol then inhibits the organism, producing a feedback shut-off of more alcohol production.

There is another example, as you know, Dr Brown. In this case sub-inhibitory concentrations of penicillin may affect adherence of streptococci to mucosal cells. This is accomplished by the effect of the antibiotic in releasing lipoteichoic acid from the bacterial cell. This substance appears responsible for attachment to cells.

Brown Sensitivity of bacteria to polymyxin requires certain kinds of phospholipids to be present in the outer membrane areas, that have an affinity for polymyxin, and therefore allow polymyxin to penetrate and damage the cytoplasmic membrane. However, with viomycin, resistance and not sensitivity is mediated by the same mechanism. The bacteria are resistant to viomycin because viomycin has an affinity to the outer membrane and certain phospholipids and is unable to penetrate the cell.

We have published a paper in the *Journal of Bacteriology* (Gilbert and Brown, 1978a) recently describing studies on chlorinated phenols. We found enhanced resistance in some cases because of the extra lipopolysaccharide on the outside of the cell which was related to growth rate and nutrient limitation. The phenol stuck to the outside of the cell and could not penetrate.

Some Biochemical Mechanisms of Antibiotics Acting Together on Bacterial Folate Metabolism

J. T. SMITH

The School of Pharmacy,
University of London, London, UK.

BACTERIAL FOLATE SYNTHESIS

Almost all medically important bacteria synthesize their dihydrofolate requirement from precursors, whereas man, who lacks this synthetic capacity, depends on preformed folates being absorbed from the diet. The absence of a dihydrofolate synthetic pathway in man makes the bacterial system vulnerable to inhibition by selective chemotherapy. However, one additional circumstance is essential before this can be accomplished. That is most, if not all, bacteria which synthesize dihydrofolate are also impermeable to exogenous folates—fortunately including those present in man (reviewed by Hitchings and Burchall, 1965).

Sulphonamides are the best known drugs which selectively inhibit the bacterial production of dihydrofolate. They prevent the condensation of a pteridine derivative (7,8-dihydro-6-hydroxymethylpterin) with *p*-aminobenzoic acid (Brown, 1962) by competitive inhibition of the enzyme dihydropteroate synthetase. The controversy over whether sulphonamides were incorporated in place of *p*-aminobenzoic acid, which they resemble, was settled by Brown (1962) who showed that such false folates are only formed in the highly artificial situation where dihydropteroate synthetase reacts with sulphonamide and the pteridine derivative in the absence of *p*-aminobenzoic acid. The final stage in the bacterial synthesis of dihydrofolate is the addition of a single molecule of glutamic acid to the dihydropteroate intermediate (Griffin and Brown, 1964) by another enzyme which could be termed dihydrofolate synthetase.

Dihydrofolic acid so synthesized by bacteria has to be further modified by reduction to tetrahydrofolate (THF) before it is of any use in bacterial metabolism. The enzyme responsible for this conversion, dihydrofolate reductase, is also present in man. However, mammalian dihydrofolate reductase differs from the bacterial enzyme in that it has the extra ability to reduce folic acid (which is the oxidized form of dihydrofolate encountered in dietary sources) to tetrahydrofolate (Hitchings and Burchall, 1965). A much more important difference from the viewpoint of selective chemotherapy is that the bacterial enzyme is very much more susceptible to inhibition by trimethoprim (Bushby and Hitchings, 1968). These differences in susceptibility are so marked that it is possible to inhibit completely the bacterial enzyme with trimethoprim at concentrations which are without effect on mammalian dihydrofolate reductase.

TETRAHYDROFOLATE METABOLISM

Tetrahydrofolate is of central importance in metabolism of both mammals and bacteria. Its role is to transfer single carbon fragments to intermediates in the syntheses of amino acids and of nuclear bases. Thus tetrahydrofolates are essential for the integrity of protein, DNA and RNA biosyntheses. Figure 1 illustrates some of the uses and the interconversions of tetrahydrofolate derivatives. It is no surprise that the abolition of this complete network of pathways has such a profound effect on bacteria when they are exposed to chemotherapy with sulphonamides or trimethoprim.

ACTION OF SULPHONAMIDES AND TRIMETHOPRIM ON BACTERIA

As stated earlier sulphonamides competitively inhibit dihydropteroate synthetase. Trimethoprim also inhibits bacterial dihydrofolate reductase in a competitive manner. Competitive inhibition, in contrast to irreversible enzymic inhibition, normally results in drugs which are merely bacteriostatic in their action. This is because under normal circumstances when such a drug is removed from the

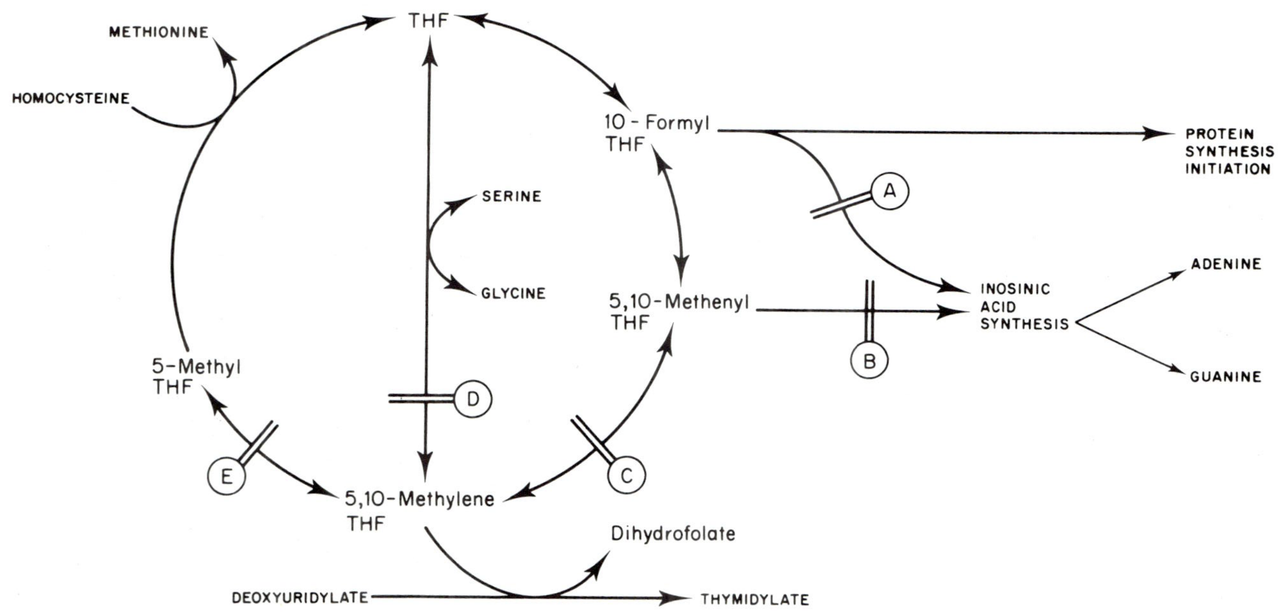
THF
METHIONINE
HOMOCYSTEINE
10 - Formyl
THF
PROTEIN
SYNTHESIS
INITIATION
SERINE
GLYCINE
A
INOSINIC
ACID
SYNTHESIS
ADENINE
GUANINE
5,10-Methenyl
THF
B
5-Methyl
THF
D
E
C
5,10-Methylene
THF
Dihydrofolate
DEOXYURIDYLATE
THYMIDYLATE

Fig. 1.

bacteria it simply diffuses away from the inhibited enzyme allowing full recovery of viability. While bacteriostasis does occur with sulphonamides or with trimethoprim both drugs can be bactericidal providing certain conditions are met.

SYNERGY BETWEEN MEDIA CONSTITUENTS AND ANTIFOLATE CHEMOTHERAPEUTIC AGENTS

Both sulphonamides and trimethoprim even in combination are merely bacteriostatic in mineral salts media (Angehrn and Then, 1973a) but when cofactors are added the action of either drug becomes bactericidal. With the two drugs combined they found that a purine such as adenine, guanine or inosine (or the equivalent purine nucleoside) together with a mixture of all the naturally occurring amino acids converted the action of the drugs to a rapid bactericidal response. Similar findings were made when sulphonamide was used singly (Then and Angehrn, 1973). With trimethoprim alone the problem was investigated in more detail and it was found that the maximum bactericidal response could still be obtained when methionine, glycine and serine were used (in place of all the amino acids) together with a purine source (Angehrn and Then, 1973b). In this paper they showed that the bactericidal response was caused by "thymineless death" (Barner and Cohen, 1954) and that when the essential cofactors were absent protein synthesis, which is essential for thymineless death, was insufficient. The synergy between media constituents and trimethoprim was studied by Amyes and Smith (1974a) who showed that a maximum bactericidal response could occur when only methionine and glycine were combined with a purine or purine nucleoside. In addition we showed that protein synthesis is required not only at the onset but also throughout the bactericidal response if maximal effect is to be obtained. Moreover, we suggested a mechanism by which these cofactors could sustain protein synthesis during trimethoprim treatment as follows.

The only tetrahydrofolate that can be oxidized to dihydrofolate is 5,10-methylene THF (Fig. 1). This uniquely occurs during the bacterial synthesis of thymidylate which is essential for DNA production. Trimethoprim which prevents re-utilization of the dihydrofolate so formed and sulphonamides which prevent even the formation of dihydrofolate thus have a deleterious effect on the bacterial supply of thymidylate. A lack of thymidylate in bacteria leads to thymineless death but this can only occur in the presence of competent protein synthesis. When any of the cofactors are absent the first pathway to be inhibited is protein synthesis and hence only bacteriostasis results.

The addition of a purine or purine nucleoside reduces the utilization of 10–formyl THF and 5,10-methenyl THF in the production of inosinic acid which is the precursor of all purine nucleotides (Fig. 1A and B). In addition purines directly interfere in the conversion of 5,10-methenyl THF to 5,10-methylene THF

(Fig. 1C). Glycine supplementation inhibits the direct formation of 5,10-methylene THF from THF and if anything should reverse this reaction in favour of THF. Methionine also inhibits the production of 5,10-methylene THF from THF (Fig. 1D) and represses the conversion of 5-methyl THF to 5,10-methylene THF (Fig. 1E). Thus the THF reserves of the bacteria are directed away from 5,10-methylene THF. This conserves 10-formyl THF which is uniquely required for initiation of the protein synthesis that is essential for a bactericidal response (Amyes and Smith, 1974a). It should be noted that not only do these cofactors act to sustain protein synthesis but also that they reduce cellular supplies of 5,10-methylene THF which must only exacerbate the lack of thymidylate synthesis in the bacteria.

These complicated interactions are not only of academic interest because synergism between methionine, glycine and a purine on the one hand and antifolate drugs on the other undoubtedly occurs *in vivo*. This became evident when Then and Angehrn (1974) showed that the cofactors essential for the bactericidal effects of trimethoprim and sulphonamides in media were also present in adequate amounts in blood and urine. Thus perhaps surprisingly both drugs which merely act by competitive inhibition initiate a series of events resulting in bacterial death. The actual cause of death during thymine starvation of bacteria remains obscure though it may possibly be caused by self-imposed DNA breakdown (Freifelder and Levine, 1972; Tweats *et al.*, 1974) which could be triggered by the absence of thymine from DNA.

SYNERGY BETWEEN TRIMETHOPRIM AND SULPHONAMIDES

There have been numerous reports on the enhanced effect that occurs when trimethoprim is used in conjunction with a sulphonamide. Obviously such studies must be made in the presence of the essential cofactors mentioned earlier. Most experiments which demonstrate synergy between the two drugs, either rely on measuring an effect which cannot be improved (for example minimum inhibitory concentrations or dose to give 50% survival (Hitchings and Burchall, 1965; Bushby and Hitchings, 1968), or observe effects at drug concentrations which cannot be measured (for example the shape of zones of inhibition around disks (Waterworth, 1969)). Both these methods hence demonstrate synergy at drug concentrations which are less than the optimal concentration of either (or both) drugs used separately. When a graded effect is measured (for example in bactericidal responses) the usual finding is that the combination cannot improve on the performance of trimethoprim, providing (i) that the latter has been tested in sufficiently high concentrations, and (ii) that the bacteria are sensitive to each separate component (see, for example, Angehrn and Then, 1973a). Thus, again, synergy can only usually be demonstrated when the amount(s) of the drugs used in the combined therapy are reduced below the concentrations necessary for optimal effect when the drugs were used singly. From these synergy studies it may seem that trimethoprim alone could be used instead of cotrimoxazole, especially as its optimal effect occurs at concentrations readily obtained in the body. This view is perhaps strengthened by the finding that the side-effects of the combination can often be ascribed to the sulphonamide component (Garrod, 1971). However, it should be noted that two provisions were made earlier. One was that trimethoprim has to be used in adequate concentrations. This condition is unlikely to be met in all instances especially in domiciliary use where patient non-compliance is common. Moreover in urinary tract infections, despite there being adequate concentrations of the drugs in the urine for uncomplicated cases there may be insufficient in the blood stream or the renal parenchyma for the cure of more complex infections like acute pyelonephritis (Brumfitt and Reeves, 1969).

The second provision mentioned earlier was that the bacteria be sensitive to each individual member of the cotrimoxazole combination. This condition is also unlikely to be fulfilled during therapy because sensitivity testing of causative organisms treated in the general practice population is not done and even in hospitals treatment may have to commence before sensitivity test results are to hand. Thus because of the high preponderance of sulphonamide resistance in hospital pathogens (Reeves, 1971) and its occurrence even in domiciliary isolates (Robertson, 1968) the chances of the bacteria being sensitive to this component are low. Trimethroprim resistance is increasing, especially in the hospital situation (Amyes *et al.*, 1978) and this further reduces the chances of the bacteria being sensitive to both components. The study of cotrimoxazole therapy by Gruneberg and Kolbe (1969) deserves mention in this context. They obtained cure rates of 93% where the causative organism was sulphonamide sensitive and 81% when it was sulphonamide resistant. These results could be taken to indicate a lack of importance of the sulphonamide moiety but equally the high cure rate in the face of resistance could suggest that synergistic interactions were taking place between the components. A recent study by Dr S. G. B. Amyes (unpublished) sheds light on resolving these opposing views. A total of 108 urinary tract isolates taken from the general practice population in Edinburgh were investigated for sensitivity to each drug and synergy in combination using a specially modified double disk technique (Amyes, 1978). Forty-four per cent of the bacteria were sensitive to both drugs, and synergy occurred with all these bacteria. Of the sulphonamide-resistant strains 43% exhibited synergy but 93% of the strains which were trimethoprim-resistant exhibited synergy. Most surprising of all was that with 36% of the bacteria resistant to both drugs synergy occurred. Thus, synergistic interactions are common despite resistance, and this factor is obviously of importance to the success of cotrimoxazole combination. It would seem unlikely that trimethoprim used singly could give such high success rates especially in those cases where bacterial antibiotic sensitivity is unknown before the commencement of therapy.

THE EMERGENCE OF RESISTANCE DURING THERAPY

On the debit side it must be pointed out that the likelihood of resistance to both components developing *during* therapy is sharply increased when resistance to one of the drugs was present *before* commencement of treatment with cotrimoxazole. This occurs clinically (Garrod, 1971) and has been demonstrated by direct experimentation (Pinney and Smith, 1973). In the latter study organisms sensitive to sulphonamide did not mutate to cotrimoxazole resistance at a detectable rate but when the same organisms were resistant to sulphonamide, cotrimoxazole resistance occurred at a high frequency. All the trimethoprim-resistant bacteria isolated in this study were found to be thymineless mutants which lack thymidylate synthetase and hence are highly resistant to trimethoprim, providing they are supplied with a thymine derivative (Amyes and Smith, 1975). This type of trimethoprim resistance occurs less commonly in clinical isolates than does trimethoprim resistance conferred by R-factors (Barker *et al.*, 1972; Okubadejo and Maskell, 1973; Amyes *et al.*, 1978). The latter type of resistance is due to the production of a highly trimethoprim-resistant R-factor-mediated dihydrofolate reductase and these bacteria resist trimethoprim without requiring a thymine source (Amyes and Smith, 1974b, 1976, 1978a). R-Factor-mediated trimethoprim resistance is thus probably more advantageous, as thymine supplies are lacking from blood and urine (Then and Angehrn, 1974). Thymine derivatives, uniquely essential for the survival of thymineless mutants, must nevertheless be present somewhere in the host or such trimethoprim-resistant bacteria would never be isolated from patients. It is possible that tissue breakdown, which probably occurs in purulent situations, would create this supply and the finding that thymineless mutants are isolated from urinary tract infections only when kidney involvement occurs supports this view (Okubadejo and Maskell, 1973).

ISOLATION OF THYMINELESS MUTANTS

One important question which must be considered in relation to the low frequencies of isolation of thymineless mutants from patients as compared with the high frequencies that are observed *in vitro* (Pinney and Smith, 1973) is: are the correct media being used? One of the factors which militates against the isolation of thymineless mutants from patients is that horse blood is often added to inferior laboratory media to "clear" them of trimethoprim and sulphonamide antagonists. Horse blood inactivates thymidine, an important antagonist of antifolate drugs, by the action of the enzyme thymidine phosphorylase which it contains (Ferone *et al.*, 1975). Unfortunately this also abolishes the ability of the medium to support the growth of thymineless mutants. In addition, media which are free from antifolate antagonists and so do not require horse blood addition have been shown to contain significant quantities of uridine or a substance acting like uridine. This was first discovered with Wellcome nutrient agar and Wellcotest agar (Amyes and Smith, 1974c). Recently we have extended this work to show that Difco Mueller Hinto Agar, Oxoid Isosensitest Agar and Wellcotest Sensitivity Test agar also suffer from the same defect (Amyes and Smith, 1978b). Uridine in these media inhibits the growth of thymineless mutants because it represses the synthesis of and inhibits preformed bacterial thymidine phosphorylase, which is the enzyme that bacteria use to assimilate exogenous thymine (Amyes and Smith, 1974c). This effect has been directly demonstrated in reconstruction experiments using mineral salts agar (Amyes and Smith, 1978c).

Thus most, if not all, laboratory media which have been "cleared" of, or to start with are free from, antagonists of antifolate chemotherapeutic agents cannot support the growth of thymineless mutants. In order for such mutants to be isolated from clinical specimens, media containing horse blood require supplementation with thymine while a medium containing uridine-like activity requires a thymidine supplement. If media contain both horse blood and uridine their use should be avoided when the isolation of thymineless mutants is desired. It is important that the actual frequency of such mutant bacteria be known so that their role in the failure of trimethoprim therapy be assessed. It should be noted that trimethoprim actually stimulates the uptake of thymine by such bacteria (Amyes and Smith, 1975) and as pointed out by Okubadejo and Maskell (1973) continued trimethoprim therapy, rather than suppressing thymineless mutants, may well maintain infection by them.

REFERENCES

Amyes, S. G. B. (1978). Synergy and Co-trimoxazole Sensitivity. *Journal of Pharmacy and Pharmacology* **30,** 13P.

Amyes, S. G. B., Emmerson, A. M. and Smith, J. T. (1978). R-factor mediated trimethoprim resistance: result of two three-month clinical surveys. *Journal of Clinical Pathology* **31,** 850–854.

Amyes, S. G. B. and Smith, J. T. (1974a). Trimethoprim action and its analogy with thymine starvation. *Antimicrobial Agents and Chemotherapy* **5,** 169–178.

Amyes, S. G. B. and Smith, J. T. (1974b). R-Factor trimethoprim resistance mechanism: an insusceptible target site. *Biochemical and Biophysical Research Communications* **58,** 412–418.

Amyes, S. G. B. and Smith, J. T. (1974c). Trimethoprim sensitivity testing and thymineless mutants. *Journal of Medical Microbiology* **7,** 143–153.

Amyes, S. G. B. and Smith, J. T. (1975). Thymineless mutants and their resistance to trimethoprim. *Journal of Antimicrobial Chemotherapy* **1,** 85–89.

Amyes, S. G. B. and Smith, J. T. (1976). The purification and properties of the trimethoprim-resistant dihydrofolate reductase mediated by the R-factor, R-388. *European Journal of Biochemistry* **61,** 597–603.

Amyes, S. G. B. and Smith, J. T. (1978a). R-Factor mediated dihydrofolate reductases which confer trimethoprim resistance. *Journal of General Microbiology* **107,** 263–271.

Amyes, S. G. B. and Smith, J. T. (1978b). Trimethoprim antagonists: effect of uridine in laboratory media. *Journal of Antimicrobial Chemotherapy* **4,** 421–429.

Amyes, S. G. B. and Smith, J. T. (1978c). Trimethoprim antagonists: effect of uridine on thymine and thymidine uptake in mineral salts medium. *Journal of Antimicrobial Chemotherapy* **4,** 415–419.

Angehrn, P. and Then, R. (1973a). Investigations into the mode of action of the combination sulphomethoxazole/trimethoprim. *Chemotherapy* **19,** 1–10.

Angehrn, P. and Then, R. (1973). Nature of trimethoprim-induced death in *E. coli. Arzneimittel Forschung* **23,** 447–451.

Barker, J., Healing, D. and Hutchison, J. G. P. (1972). Characteristics of some cotrimoxazole resistant Enterobacteriaceae from infected patients. *Journal of Clinical Pathology* **25,** 1086–1088.

Barner, H. D. and Cohen, S. S. (1954). The induction of thymine synthesis by T2 infection of a thymine requiring mutant of *E. coli. Journal of Bacteriology* **68,** 80–88.

Brown, G. M. (1962). The biosynthesis of folic acid. Inhibition by sulphonamides. *Journal of Biological Chemistry* **237,** 536–540.

Brumfitt, W. and Reeves, D. S. (1969). Recent developments in the treatment of urinary tract infections. *Journal of Infectious Diseases* **120,** 61–81.

Bushby, S. R. M. and Hitchings, G. H. (1968). Trimethoprim, a sulphonamide potentiator. *British Journal of Pharmacology and Chemotherapy* **33,** 72–90.

Ferone, R., Bushby, S. R. M., Burchall, J. J., Moore, W. D. and Smith, D. (1975). Identification of Harper–Cawston Factor as thymidine phosphorylase and removal from media of substances interfering with susceptibility testing to sulphonamides and diaminopyrimidines. *Antimicrobial Agents and Chemotherapy* **7,** 91–98.

Freifelder, D. and Levine, E. (1972). Stimulation of nuclease activity by thymine starvation. *Biochemical and Biophysical Research Communications* **46,** 1782–1787.

Garrod, L. P. (1971). Trimethoprim: its possible place in antibacterial therapy. *Drugs* **1,** 3–53.

Griffin, M. J. and Brown, G. M. (1964). The Biosynthesis of folic acid III. *Journal of Biological Chemistry* **239,** 310–316.

Gruneberg, R. N. and Kolbe, R. (1969). Trimethoprim in the treatment of urinary infections in hospital. *British Medical Journal* **1,** 545–547.

Hitchings, G. H. and Burchall, J. J. (1965). Inhibition of folate biosynthesis and function as a basis for chemotherapy. *Advances in Enzymology* **27,** 417–468.

Okubadejo, O. A. and Maskell, R. M. (1973). Thymine-requiring mutants of *Proteus mirabilis* selected by cotrimoxazole *in vivo*. *Journal of General Microbiology* **77,** 533–535.

Pinney, R. J. and Smith, J. T. (1973). Joint trimethoprim and sulphamethoxazole resistance in bacteria infected with R-factors. *Journal of Medical Microbiology* **6,** 13–19.

Reeves, D. S. (1971). Sulphamethoxazole/trimethoprim: the first two years. *Journal of Clinical Pathology* **24,** 430–437.

Robertson, M. H. (1968). Antibiotic resistance patterns of organisms causing acute urinary tract infections occurring in general practice. *British Journal of Clinical Practice* **22,** 63–67.

Then, R. and Angehrn, P. (1973). Sulphonamide-induced thymineless death in *E. coli. Journal of General Microbiology* **76,** 255–263.

Then, R. and Angehrn, P. (1974). The biochemical basis of antimicrobial action of sul-

phonamides and trimethoprim *in vivo*. *Biochemical Pharmacology* **23,** 2977–2982.
Tweats, D. J., Pinney, R. J. and Smith, J. T. (1974). R-factor-mediated nuclease activity involved in thymineless elimination. *Journal of Bacteriology* **118,** 790–795.
Waterworth, P. M. (1969). Practical aspects of testing sensitivity to trimethoprim and sulphonamide. *Postgraduate Medical Journal* **45,** Suppl. 21–29.

DISCUSSION

Brumfitt This is a demonstration of a piece of highly capable work which doesn't seem to correlate the clinical findings. Professor Asscher and I have been involved in a large multi-centre trial in Cardiff, Bath and London and the fact of the matter is we have not had a problem with antibiotic resistance.

We have been looking at all the bacterial isolates at the Royal Free Hospital over the last three years and the paper reporting this is in the press.

Your findings of thymineless mutants is interesting because we didn't find any during the three year period. R-Factor-resistance which you considered common is, I think, very rare; we have succeeded in finding eleven. I gather that Dr Datta's series added up to ten, one of which came from a cow.

Smith I said, "The R-factor mechanism is very rare but even so its occurrence is more common than the finding of thymineless mutants".

Brumfitt If resistance does occur it is chromosomally mediated and we have found this to be due to a type of dihydrofolate reductase which has much lower affinity for trimethoprim. It is excessively rare in *E. coli*—only 3% of the proven urine infections—and this resistance is in the range of 4–600 $\mu g\ ml^{-1}$. And of the 3%, 65% were totally resistant. So it looks as though these organisms are the ones that are going to cause trouble.

One other thing that causes me great alarm is the reporting of sensitivity, because people are reporting trimethoprim resistance on the basis of finding that the organisms resisted sulphonamide or trimethoprim. This is very strange thinking. This is one of the major problems caused by people spreading pus on plates and doing direct testing. At the present time there isn't any reason to fear. When we did the first trial on cotrimoxazole I urged the companies to market trimethoprim alone and for scientific reasons (mainly the fear of resistance and because of the synergy) they decided not to do this. We did a trial in 1960 where we compared cotrimoxazole, trimethoprim, ampicillin and cephalosporin. Even then the results between cotrimoxazole and trimethoprim were the same.

Smith I quite agree with every word you have said because what you are talking about is urinary tract infections and I said this morning (and Dr Greenwood said it as well) that in such infections the sulphonamide contribution is not of too much importance. What I am talking about is in every type of infection we cannot be too complacent of using trimethoprim on its own. We know that the thymineless mutant mutation rate is high and it would stop any trimethoprim therapy from working in infections where there are thymine and thymidine supplies, and in these cases I believe the sulphonamide contribution in cotrimoxazole is important in therapy.

One other point is that all the Wellcome media contain a uridine-like substance which prevents the growth of thymineless mutants on them. Thus the frequency of isolation of thymineless mutants on these media is much less than the true frequency of their occurrence.

Greenwood I would like to raise three points. First, going back to your unfavourable remarks about turbidimetry compared with viable counting, we reached the same conclusions about trimethoprim–sulphonamide synergy by turbidimetric methods as you did by viable counting. Turbidimetry is a much less laborious technique than viable counting and it gives a continuous record over an extended time scale. So turbidimetry, if used sensibly, and combined with microscopy is a very useful method.

My second point is about the emergence of spontaneous resistance to trimethoprim. One reason why spontaneous resistance emerges frequently *in vitro* is because selecting for resistance is made at 4 μg trimethoprim per ml, which is just above the normal MIC.

My last point is that if you are saying the emergence of spontaneous resistance during treatment is not a problem, but resistance in an ecological sense might be important, then you have abandoned the concept of using these two agents—trimethoprim and sulphonamide—in any biochemically interactive way. You are merely using two antibiotics to prevent the emergence of resistance.

Smith That's not a bad thing.

Greenwood But there is no reason why sulphonamide should be the partner of trimethoprim in this case.

Smith We haven't done experiments with other compounds, but we know sulphonamide stops trimethoprim resistance emerging.

Acar I would like to ask about the data in which the synergistic effects are presented (p.92). Either the strains are sulphonamide resistant or trimethoprim resistant? What are the species studied? Have you any data relating the mechanism of the resistance to the presence or absence of a synergistic activity between the two drugs?

Smith They were all gram-negative rods and nearly all were *E. coli*. The mechanism of resistance has not been fully worked out except that two had R-factors. None were found to be thymineless mutants. The majority are resistant either because they are impermeable or because they have got elevated dihydrofolate reductase levels; and in some cases they have a resistant dihydrofolate reductase.

We thought it would be useful if one could test for synergy and say, "there is synergy when the mechanism of resistance is A" and say, "no synergy when the mechanism of resistance is B". However, we found you cannot predict the mechanism of resistance from observations of synergy. With the R-factor-mediated mechanism there is synergy if there is a small amount of enzyme, but if the level of enzyme is high there is no synergy.

Acar In a similar study among 100 strains of *E. coli* which were sulphonamide resistant, 78 showed a synergistic activity between sulphonamide and trimethoprim.

Inhibitors of Antibiotic-Inactivating Enzymes

M. COLE

Beecham Pharmaceuticals, Research Division,
Betchworth, Surrey, UK.

INTRODUCTION

Enzymic transformation of certain antibiotics into compounds with little or no antibacterial activity is a well established resistance mechanism in certain strains of bacteria. Chloramphenicol can be inactivated by *O*-acetylation or *N*-deacetylation, aminoglycosides by *N*-acetylation, *O*-phosphorylation and *O*-adenylylation, and penicillins and cephalosporins by β-lactamase hydrolysis of the β-lactam ring or enzymic deacylation of the side chain. Only in the case of β-lactamase has inhibition been extensively studied and applied to the enhancement of the antibacterial activity of labile penicillins and cephalosporins. Although certain aminoglycosides have been reported to inhibit specific aminoglycoside-inactivated enzymes, the large number of sites of attack has probably impeded the selection and application of suitable inhibitors. On the other hand, the availability of a wide range of structural variants of penicillins and cephalosporins, including compounds stable to β-lactamase, has encouraged research on inhibitors of β-lactamase although the existence of a great variety of β-lactamases is a problem.

The role of these β-lactamases in the cell is still the subject of debate, but it is certain that they are frequently associated with the resistance of bacterial cells to both penicillins and cephalosporins (Sykes and Matthew, 1976). The low toxicity shown by penicillins and cephalosporins has encouraged the search for derivatives which are stable to β-lactamase and thereby effective against resistant strains of bacteria. The penicillins methicillin and cloxacillin (Nayler *et al.*, 1962) and the cephalosporin derivatives cefoxitin and cefuroxime (Richmond and Wotton, 1976) are examples of compounds of this type. However, it has proved difficult to find derivatives with complete stability to a wide range of β-lactamases without sacrificing some antibacterial activity. This has encouraged an alternative approach to the problem of β-lactamase-based resistance, namely the use of β-lactamase inhibitors to mitigate the destructive effect of the enzyme.

The main types of inhibitors of antibiotic-inactivating enzymes are described below in the context of their application as antibacterial synergists.

CHLORAMPHENICOL AND AMINOGLYCOSIDE-INACTIVATING ENZYMES

Chloramphenicol-resistant strains can inactivate chloramphenicol by enzymic removal of the chloracetyl group (Vining, 1975) or by acetylation of the hydroxyl groups (Davies and Rownd, 1972; Shaw, 1975) (Fig. 1), but inhibition of these enzymes by compounds other than non-specific enzyme inactivating agents has not been reported.

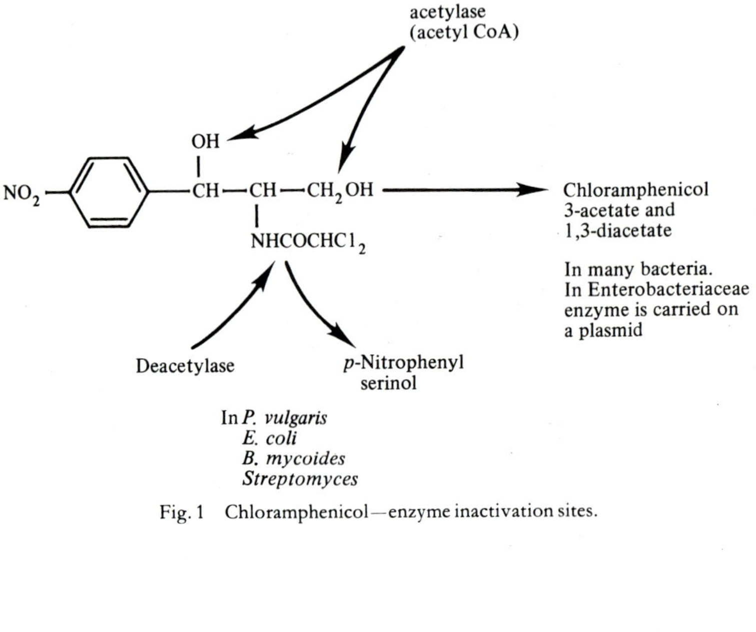

Fig. 1 Chloramphenicol—enzyme inactivation sites.

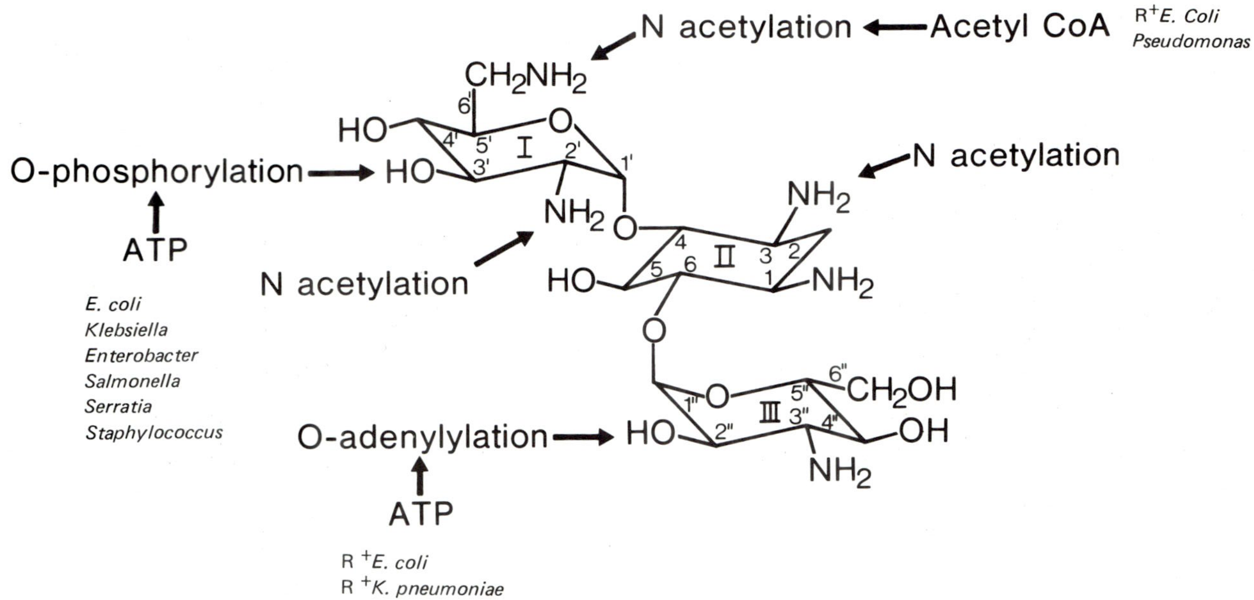

Fig. 2 Kanamycin B—enzyme inactivation sites.

The mechanism of resistance to the various aminoglycoside antibiotics has been extensively investigated. Three types of enzymic systems have been discovered, namely phosphorylation and adenylylation of hydroxy groups and acetylation of amino groups. These reactions lead to a reduction or elimination of antibacterial activity and are found in strains of bacteria carrying resistance (R) factors (Benveniste and Davies, 1973; Haas and Dowding, 1975). All of these reactions have been found to occur for the kanamycin family of aminoglycosides, as shown in Fig. 2 for kanamycin B. Benveniste and Davies (1973) list three different acetylating enzymes, four phosphorylating enzymes and two adenylylating enzymes as being produced by various bacteria.

Chemical modification of various groups in the aminoglycoside structure has enabled compounds to be made which are no longer substrates for certain inactivating enzymes, thus the acylation of the 1-amino group of the middle ring system of kanamycin with 1-L-hydroxy-3-aminobutyric acid gave amikacin. This compound has a broader antibacterial spectrum, being stable to 3′-*O*-phosphorylation, 2″-*O*-adenylation and 3-*N*-acetylation (Kawaguchi, 1977) but is still a substrate for *N*-acetylation at the 6 amino position of ring I (Price *et al.*, 1974; Yagisawa *et al.*, 1975). Members of the gentamicin group of aminoglycosides are also inactivated by enzymes produced by R-factor-carrying strains of resistant bacteria, acetylation and adenylylation being involved. Modification of this structure by *N*-ethylation at position 1 of ring II and introduction of a double bond at the 4′-5′-position of ring I gives netilmicin, a compound with improved stability (Kawaguchi, 1977).

INHIBITION OF AMINOGLYCOSIDE-INACTIVATING ENZYMES

Little work has been published on the inhibition of these enzymes but Benveniste and Davies (1971) have reported the specific inhibition of the *N*-acetylation at the 6′ position of kanamycin A and gentamicin C_{1a} by other non-substrate aminoglycosides having no amino group in the 6′-position as shown in Table I. At equimolar concentrations (about 0·2 mM) up to 80% inhibition was observed by what appears to be a competitive inhibition reaction, judging by the fact that the percentage inhibition did not change when the enzyme and inhibitor were preincubated. The products formed by *N*-acetylation of kanamycin A and gentamicin C_{1a} were poor inhibitors of the acetylation reaction. The structural relationship between a substrate such as gentamicin C_{1a} and an inhibitor such as gentamicin A is shown in Fig. 3. Yagisawa *et al.* (1975) reported substrate inhibition of 6′-acetylation at concentrations above 83 μM for kanamycin B, amikacin and tobramycin. Kanamycin C and paromamine which did not have the 6′-amino group were non-competitive inhibitors with K_i values of 8·3 and $69{\cdot}8 \times 10^{-6}$M respectively.

TABLE I.

Inhibition of the aminoglycoside *N*-acetylating enzyme produced by *E. coli* W677 carrying R factor R5. (From Benveniste and Davies, 1971.)

Inhibitor*	Inhibition of acetylation (%)	
	Kanamycin A†	Gentamicin C_{1a}
Gentamicin A	64	81
Gentamicin C_1	10	9
Paromomycin	76	80
Paromamine (= gentamine A, not an antibiotic)	41	43
N-Acetyl kanamycin A	0	—
N-Acetyl gentamicin C_{1a}	—	30

* Equimolar with substrate.
† Product of *N*-acetylation of Kanamycin A is antibacterially inactive and that of Gentamicin C_{1a} reduced is in activity.

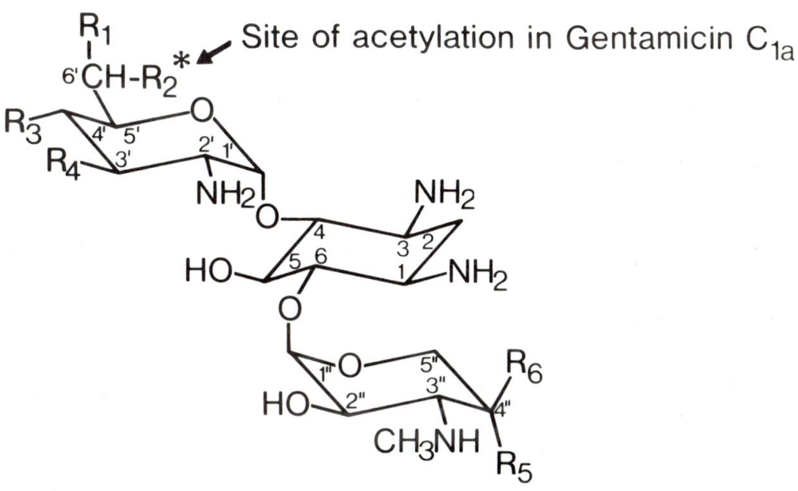

	R_1	R_2	R_3	R_4	R_5	R_6
Gentamicin C_{1a} (substrate)	H	NH_2*	H	H	OH	CH_3
Gentamicin A (inhibitor)	H	OH	OH	OH	H	OH

Fig. 3 Structural features of a substrate and an inhibitor of the aminoglycoside acetylating enzyme of *E. coli* W677 R5 (from Benveniste and Davis, 1971).

Umezawa (1970) has described the inhibition of kanamycin 3′-hydroxy phosphorylation. As this reaction requires magnesium ions it is probably not surprising that EDTA was found to be an inhibitor. The reaction also requires ATP as phosphate donor and ADP, AMP and adenosine at 3·2 mM were found to be good inhibitors. The only inhibitor with a structural relationship to the substrate was methyl 3-amino-3-deoxy-α-D-glucopyranoside (67% inhibition at 3·2 mM), the inhibition being competitive. According to Davies and Rownd (1972), compounds lacking the 3′-hydroxy substituent inhibit phosphorylation if otherwise similar in structure. For example, gentamicin C_{1a}, tobramycin and sisomicin inhibit kanamycin phosphotransferase.

Interestingly, Benveniste and Davies (1971) speculate that in clinical use the gentamicin complex may have some advantage over the use of the individual components since it contains inhibitors of the acetylation and phosphorylation reactions.

The existence of so many different types of aminoglycoside-inactivating enzymes is a major obstacle to the selection of an inhibitor of these enzymes. However, for aminoglycosides having only one major site of enzymic inactivation the selection of an effective inhibitor may be possible.

PENICILLIN- AND CEPHALOSPORIN-INACTIVATING ENZYMES

The most important enzyme inactivation process responsible for resistance to penicillins, involves the hydrolysis of the β-lactam ring by β-lactamase to give antibacterially inactive penicilloic acid. Strains of bacteria showing high resistance to penicillins usually produce β-lactamase but permeability barriers can also exist (Sykes and Matthew, 1976). The antibacterial activity of penicillins can also be reduced by enzymic removal of the side chain by deacylase enzymes to give 6-aminopenicillanic acid. However, this latter reaction is not an important resistance mechanism (Cole and Sutherland, 1966).

Hydrolysis of the β-lactam ring in cephalosporins is also the most important enzymic route by which these compounds are rendered inactive against resistant strains, although again permeability barriers may play a part. This reaction usually proceeds to give further degradation products, rather than cephalosporoic acid. The enzymic removal of the side chain to give 7-aminocephalosporanic acid can also take place but has not been reported to be associated with a resistance mechanism. The enzymic removal of the acetyl group from cephalosporins containing the 3-acetoxymethyl substituent can occur in the body to give deacetyl cephalosporin of reduced antibacterial activity (O'Callaghan and Muggleton, 1963). This reaction has also been found to be carried out by various microorganisms (Demain *et al.*, 1963; Abbott and Fukuda, 1975) but has not been reported to be an important resistance mechanism in bacteria.

Several different types of β-lactamase inhibitor have been reported and have been reviewed (Cole, 1979). Examples of the more important types are discussed below in relation to their use as agents to enhance the activity of labile β-lactam antibiotics against bacteria resistant by virtue of β-lactamase production. Inhibitors of the side chain deacylase enzymes have also been reported, for example the products of the reaction (Savidge and Cole, 1975), but have not been investigated in such detail as β-lactamase inhibitors and have not been shown to enhance the antibacterial activity of penicillins against resistant strains. The various sites of enzymic attack on penicillins and cephalosporins leading to reduction or elimination of antibacterial activity are shown in Figure 4.

A wide variety of microorganisms produce β-lactamase and mammalian forms of the enzyme seem to exist (Table II). There are many different types of β-lactamase, the characteristics and classification of which have been extensively reviewed (Richmond and Sykes, 1973; Sykes and Matthew, 1976). Although substrate profiles can distinguish many of the different types of enzyme, isoelectric focusing on ultrasonicated cell extracts is now used for rapid preliminary characterization (Matthew *et al.*, 1975). Figure 5 is a photograph of the isoelectric

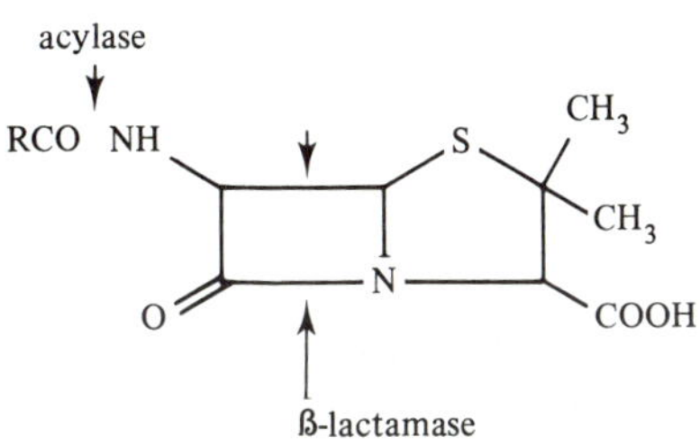

Penicillins

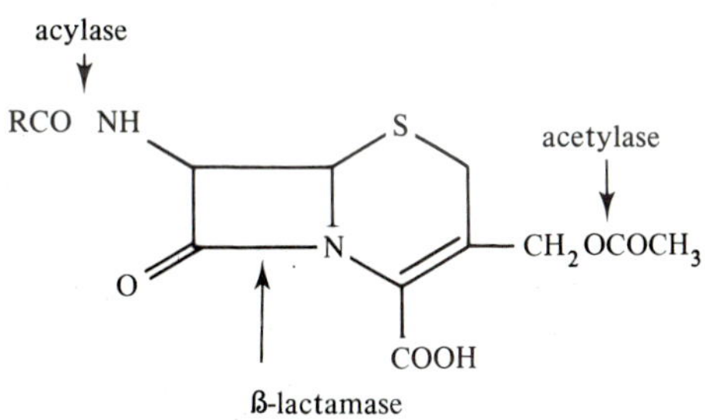

Cephalosporins

Fig. 4 Points of enzymic attack on penicillins and cephalosporins.

TABLE II.

Occurrence of ß-lactamase.

Type of activity	Source	References
	Micro-organisms	
Hydrolysis of penicillins and/or cephalosporins	Many strains of bacteria including *Staph. aureus, B. cereus, P. mirabilis, K. aerogenes, E. coli, Ps. aeruginosa, Ent. cloacae*	Citri and Pollock (1966); Richmond and Sykes (1973); Sykes and Matthew (1976)
	Streptomyces species	Johnson *et al.* (1975); Ogawara *et al.* (1978a, b)
	Moulds	Citri and Pollock (1966)
	Candida albicans	Mehta and Nash (1978)
	Blue-green algae	Kushner *et al.* (1977)
	D-Alanine carboxypeptidases	
Weak penicillinase	*E. coli* H2143	Tamura *et al.* (1976)
ß-Lactam ring cleaved at CO-N bond and 5,6-carbon bonds; phenylacetylglycine liberated	*Streptomyces* R61 *Bacillus stearothermophilus*	Frère *et al.* (1976); Hammarström and Strominger (1976)
	Mammals	
Inactivation of benzylpenicillin methyl ester	Plasma and liver —guinea-pig, mouse and rabbit	Snow (1962)
Inactivation of penicillins	Liver —rat	Kind *et al.* (1968)
Inactivation of chromogenic cephalosporin	Serum	O'Callaghan (1978)
Penicilloic acid excreted	Man	Cole *et al.* (1973); Graber *et al.* (1976)

focusing patterns for the ß-lactamases used to obtain the enzyme inhibition profiles shown in the tables which follow. The isoelectric focusing was carried out in polyacrylamide–ampholine gel to which starch was added. Zones of enzyme activity were located by flooding the gel plates with a solution containing benzylpenicillin, KI and iodine to reveal white zones of penicilloic acid on a dark blue background.

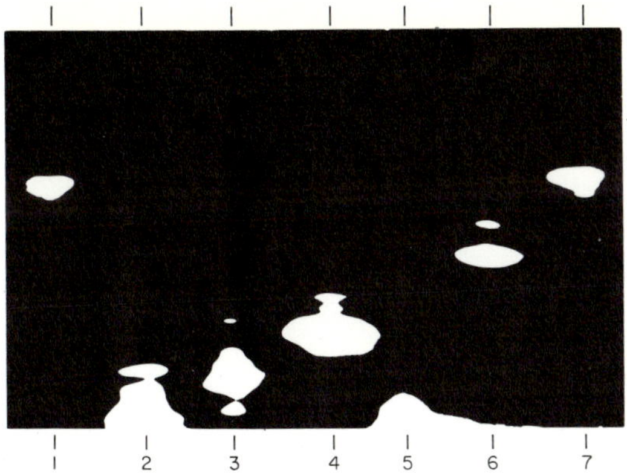

1. *E. coli* K12 R^+TEM
2. *E. coli* JT 414
3. *Ps. aeruginosa*
4. *K. pneumoniae* ATCC 29665
5. *Ent. cloacae* NCTC 10005
6. *P. mirabilis* C 889
7. *E. coli* K12 R^+TEM

Fig. 5 Isoelectric focusing patterns of β-lactamases.

The association between the ability to produce β-lactamase and resistance to penicillin is illustrated in Table III for *Staphylococcus aureus*. The effect of using the β-lactamase-stable penicillin, methicillin, is also illustrated. It can be clearly seen that although methicillin has similar activity against penicillinase-positive and -negative strains of *Staph. aureus*, its activity is much less than that of benzylpenicillin against the penicillinase-negative strain. In other words, activity has been sacrificed in obtaining a compound with improved stability to β-lactamase. The attraction of looking for inhibitors of β-lactamase thus stems from the possibility of being able to make labile β-lactam antibiotics as active against resistant strains as against sensitive ones.

TABLE III.

Effect of β-lactamase production on the activity of penicillins against *Staphylococcus aureus*. (From Rolinson and Sutherland, 1973.)

Penicillin	Minimum inhibitory concentration ($\mu g\ ml^{-1}$) β-lactamase-negative strain	β-lactamase-positive strain
Benzylpenicillin	0·02	> 250
Methicillin	1·25	2·5

Early Work on β-lactamase Inhibitors

The interest in inhibition of penicillinase started a very long time ago. Examples of the kind of results obtained are shown in Table IV, together with references to the first observations of inhibitory activity in β-lactam antibiotics, namely cephalosporin C and methicillin.

TABLE IV.

Penicillinase inhibitors—early literature.

Material	Inhibition	Enzyme	Antibacterial synergy	Reference
Antipenicillinase serum	+ve	penicillinase	No data	Perlstein and Liebmann (1945)
Na-Laurylsulphate	+ve	clarase and *E. coli*	No data	Reid *et al.* (1946)
Pepsin and papain	50–95%	*B. cereus*	No data	Henry and Housewright (1947)
Sulphonamides (suspension)	+ve	penicillinase	No data	Cronheim *et al.* (1949)
2-Benzylimidazole D-Penicillamine	+ve ±ve	penicillinase penicillinase	±ve +ve (*B. cereus*)	Behrens and Garrison (1950)
Xylocaine	+ve	*Staph. aureus*	+ve (*Staph.*)	Vaczi and Uri (1954)
Antipenicillinase serum	+ve	penicillinase	(*Staph.*) ±ve	Tacking (1955)
Cephalosporin C	I_{50} 8mM	*B. cereus*	No data	Abraham and Newton (1956)
Methicillin	90%	*B. cereus*	No data	Rolinson *et al.* (1960)

PENICILLINS AND CEPHALOSPORINS AS INHIBITORS OF β-LACTAMASE

Table V illustrates the β-lactamase inhibitory properties of the antistaphylococcal penicillins methicillin and cloxacillin, which were the first penicillins to be found to have significant β-lactamase inhibitory activity (Jago *et al.*, 1963; Hamilton-Miller, 1963; Sutherland and Batchelor, 1964). The profound effect which the structure of the side chain has on the inhibition profile can be seen. The attach-

TABLE V.

β-Lactamase inhibitory activity of cloxacillin, methicillin, carbenicillin, cephalothin and cephoxazole. (From Beecham Pharmaceuticals, unpublished data.)

Source of *β*-lactamase	Percentage inhibition by compound at 40 μg ml^{-1}—benzylpenicillin substrate at 1 mg ml^{-1}				
	Penicillins X = 6APA			Cephalosporins Y = 7ACA	
	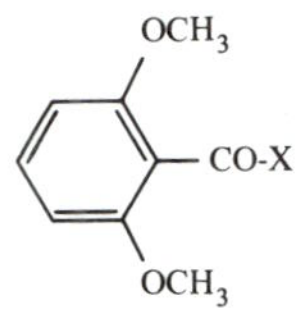	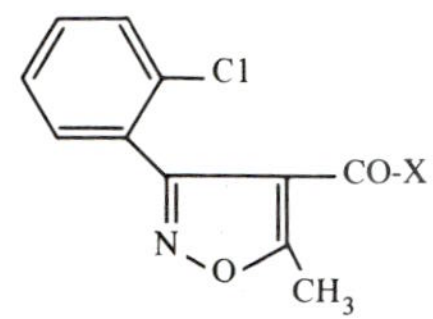	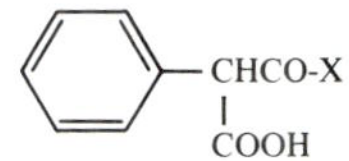	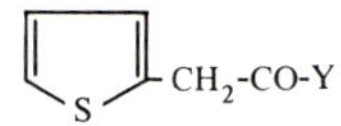	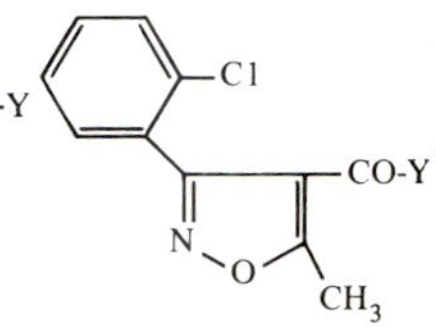
	Methicillin	Cloxacillin	Carbenicillin	Cephalothin	Cephoxazole
E. coli K12 R TEM	62 (24)*	3	0	11	0
E. coli JT 414	67 (18)	96 (0·14)	100 (0·9)	17	100 (4)
P. mirabilis C889	21	33	0	8	0
K. aerogenes A NCTC 418	100 (2·5)	10	15	12	94 (11)
Ent. cloacae NCTC 10005	5	95 (2·5)	100 (1·9)	3	100 (0·9)
Ps. aeruginosa A	73 (7·5)	87 (2·2)	81 (14)	2	100 (0·4)
Staph. aureus MB9	0	2	0	75 (10)	0

* I_{50} values—concentration (μg ml^{-1}) required to give 50% inhibition with benzylpenicillin as substrate at 1 mg ml^{-1}.

ment of the cloxacillin side chain to the cephalosporin nucleus gives an inhibitor with somewhat broader inhibition profile. The inhibitory activity of this compound, which was called cephoxazole, was first described by O'Callaghan and Morris (1972). The inhibition profile for the cephalosporin cephalothin is quite different from that for the other compounds in that it only inhibits the staphylococcal enzyme. Methicillin and cloxacillin have also been shown to inhibit staphylococcal β-lactamase but only at very high concentrations (for references see Cole, 1979). Carbenicillin has been reported to have β-lactamase inhibitory activity (Zemelman and Olivari, 1972; Labia *et al.*, 1974) and, as can be seen from Table V, has an inhibition profile not unlike cloxacillin. The cephalosporin corresponding to carbenicillin, i.e. with the α-carboxybenzyl side chain, also has β-lactamase inhibitory activity while its 7-methoxy derivative is a very potent inhibitor of the β-lactamase of *Enterobacter cloacae* (Mahoney *et al.*, 1976). A new, β-lactamase-stable, highly active cephalosporin, HR 756 (cefotaxime), has been claimed to have high inhibitory activity against the β-lactamases of *Citrobacter* and *Proteus morganii* with K_i values of $7{\cdot}7 \times 10^{-3}$ μM and $1{\cdot}2 \times 10^{-2}$ μM (Fu and Neu, 1978).

The ability of the β-lactamase inhibitor cloxacillin to protect ampicillin from destruction, thereby rendering it active against certain ampicillin-resistant strains of gram-negative bacteria, *in vitro* and *in vivo* is illustrated in Table VI (Sutherland, 1977). Figure 6 shows the results for the effect of ampicillin alone or ampicillin combined with cloxacillin on the rate of growth of a culture of *Proteus morganii* (Acred and Sutherland, 1967). The results illustrate that the effect of cloxacillin is to prevent the destruction of the ampicillin, thereby maintaining its concentration at a sufficient level to sterilize the culture. In other words, the synergistic effect seen between ampicillin and cloxacillin is attributable to the inhibition of the β-lactamase. Cloxacillin was reported to give an I_{50} value of $0{\cdot}2\,\mu g\,ml^{-1}$ against the β-lactamase of *P. morganii* G when using $1\,mg\,ml^{-1}$ benzylpenicillin as substrate (Hamilton-Miller and Smith, 1964).

TABLE VI.

Synergistic activity of ampicillin with cloxacillin against ampicillin resistant bacteria, *in vitro* and *in vivo*. (From Sutherland, 1977.)

	MIC ($\mu g\,ml^{-1}$) in agar			CD_{50}* ($mg\,kg^{-1}$)—oral		
	Amp.	Clox.	Amp. + Clox.	Amp.	Clox.	Amp. + Clox.
E. coli	250	500	25 + 25	>5 000	>1 000	320 + 320
Shigella sonnei	250	500	12·5 + 12·5	>5 000	>1 000	90 + 90
Proteus morganii	125	1 000	12·5 + 12·5	>5 000	>1 000	80 + 80

*Mice infected i.p. and dosed immediately after injection with a single dose of the compound or combination.

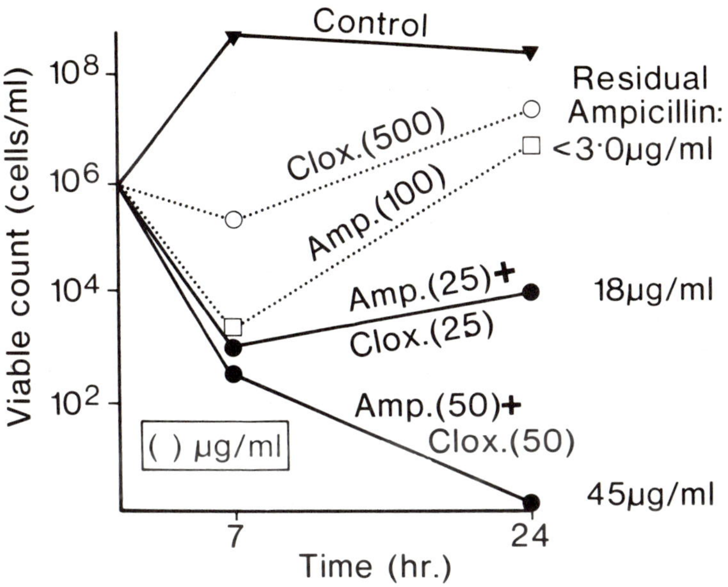

Fig. 6 Potentiation of the bactericidal activity of ampicillin against *Proteus morganii* by inhibition of its β-lactamase by cloxacillin (from Acred and Sutherland, 1967).

Various isoxazolyl penicillins are available in formulations with ampicillin or amoxycillin, and cephoxazole formulated with benzylpenicillin has recently been made available for veterinary application. These mixtures may, in certain instances, have greater antibacterial activity than the additive effects of the components by virtue of the protective effect of the β-lactamase inhibitor.

The discovery of the β-lactamase inhibitory activity of methicillin stimulated the investigation of other alkoxy substituted penicillins (Table VII) and led to the selection of the potent β-lactamase inhibitor 2-isopropoxy-1-naphthyl penicillin (BRL 1437) (Cole *et al.*, 1972). The related penicillin 2-ethoxy-1-naphthyl penicillin (nafcillin) is also a very active β-lactamase inhibitor (O'Callaghan and Morris, 1972; Cole *et al.*, 1972). Nafcillin is stable to staphylococcal β-lactamase and is clinically available for treating penicillin resistant staphylococci. The β-lactamase inhibition profile for BRL 1437 is shown in Table VIII. BRL 1437 has potent inhibitory activity against R_{TEM} and *K. aerogenes* β-lactamases and is a competitive inhibitor of these enzymes, the inhibitory activity being little affected by prior incubation with β-lactamase. BRL 1437 has very high stability to *E. coli* β-lactamase compared with cloxacillin and methicillin. The K_i values of 4×10^{-3} µM and 1×10^{-3} µM were reported for the β-lactamases of *E. coli* B11 and *K. aerogenes* A respectively (Cole *et al.*, 1972).

TABLE VII.

Alkoxynaphthyl penicillins as inhibitors of the β-lactamase of *E. coli* B11. (From Cole *et al.*, 1972.)

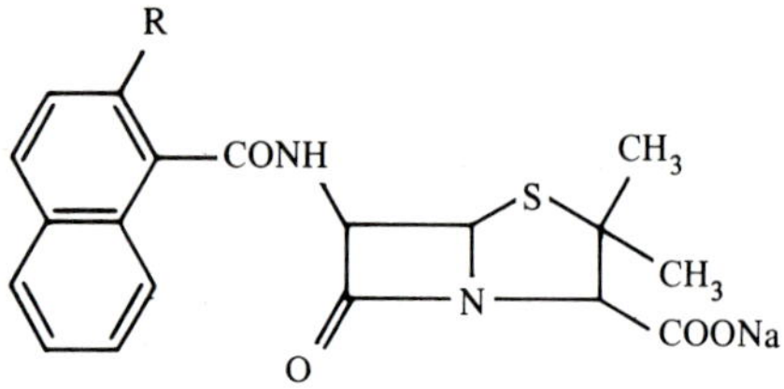

BRL Compound No.	R	K_i value (μM)
1371	—H	a substrate
1336	$—OCH_3$	0·24
1383*	$—OCH_2CH_3$	0·028
1389	$—OCH_2CH_2CH_3$	0·019
1437	$—OCH<^{CH_3}_{CH_3}$	0·004
1396	$—OCH_2CH_2CH_2CH_3$	0·016
1241	Methicillin	0·29

* Nafcillin.

The potentiating effect of BRL 1437 on the antibacterial activity of ampicillin and cephalothin against a variety of gram-negative bacteria is illustrated in Table IX (Beecham British Patent 1 460 577). Improved efficacy of BRL 1437 in combination with a cephalosporin, compared with ampicillin, is seen. A concentration of 20 μg ml^{-1} BRL 1437 was not very effective at lowering the MIC of ampicillin, but was effective at lowering the MIC of cephalothin. As BRL 1437 is a competitive inhibitor its effectiveness will be influenced by the affinity of the labile substrate for the enzyme. As cephalothin has a lower affinity than ampicillin for the β-lactamase, this may at least be part of the explanation why better results are obtained with cephalothin.

Methicillin was the first penicillin to be used clinically as a β-lactamase inhibitor. Shirley and Moore (1965) described the successful treatment of a *Pseudomonas aeruginosa* urinary tract infection using methicillin in combination with benzylpenicillin. Since this time many papers have been published describing antibacterial synergy between β-lactamase inhibitors such as methicillin, nafcillin, cloxacillin, dicloxacillin, flucloxacillin and β-lactamase-labile compounds such as ampicillin and cephaloridine. These results have been reviewed by Cole (1979). In most cases the concentration of inhibitor required to give good antibacterial synergy was much higher than readily achieved in blood but often within the range obtained in urine, suggesting that such mixtures may be of use in treating urinary tract infections.

MISCELLANEOUS INHIBITORS OF β-LACTAMASE

Certain compounds with structures resembling the penicillin molecule have been described as having weak or narrow spectrum inhibitory activity. The structures and properties of these compounds have been reviewed (Cole, 1979) but the most notable is 3(*p*-nitrophenylacetamido)-4-phenyl-2-azetidinone which inhibits staphylococcal β-lactamase and enhances the antibacterial activity of benzylpenicillin against β-lactamase-producing staphylococci.

TABLE VIII.

β-Lactamase inhibitory activity of BRL 1437 (2-isopropoxy-1-naphthylpenicillin). (From Beecham Pharmaceuticals, unpublished data.)

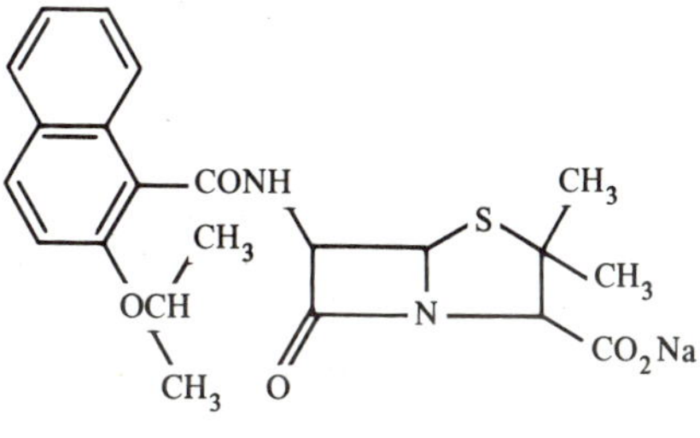

Source of β-lactamase	I_{50} values (μg ml^{-1}) Substrate* added immediately after inhibitor	Substrate* added 15 min. after inhibitor
E. coli K12 R TEM	0·18	0·21
E. coli JT 414	18	16
P. mirabilis C889	34	13
K. aerogenes A	0·78	0·88
Ent. cloacae NCTC 10005	9	4
Ps. aeruginosa A	22	14
Staph. aureus MB9	—	>40

* Substrate: benzylpenicillin 1 mg ml^{-1}.

TABLE IX.

Synergism between the β-lactamase inhibitor BRL 1437 and ampicillin or cephalothin (Beecham British Patent 1 460 577).

Organism		Minimum inhibitory concentrations (in agar) ($\mu g\ ml^{-1}$)			
		Ampicillin alone	Ampicillin + $20\ \mu g\ ml^{-1}$ BRL 1437*	Cephalothin alone	Cephalothin + $20\ \mu g\ ml^{-}_{1}$ BRL 1437*
E. coli	54	250	50	1 000	5
	6	250	100	>1 000	25
	61	1 000	250	10	2·5
	7	>1 000	500	25	5
K. aerogenes	3	250	50	5	<5
	37	>1 000	500	25	<5
	29	>1 000	1 000	50	12·5
	52	>1 000	>1 000	250	50

* MIC values for BRL 1437 = $250\ \mu g\ ml^{-1}$ or greater.

NATURALLY OCCURRING β-LACTAMASE INHIBITORS

The first reference to the possible existence of a naturally occurring β-lactamase inhibitor is in a paper by Hutter and Welsch (1948). These authors describe the production by *Penicillium notatum* of an "antipenicillinase" factor which reduced the rate of hydrolysis of benzylpenicillin by actinomycete penicillinase. The chemical nature of this factor was not established. The first naturally occurring, highly active β-lactamase inhibitor to be fully characterized was clavulanic acid. This substance is produced by *Streptomyces clavuligerus* ATCC 27064 and was detected by testing culture filtrates for β-lactamase inhibitory activity (Brown *et al.*, 1976; Reading and Cole, 1977). Elucidation of its structure revealed that it had a bicyclic ring system resembling the nucleus of the penicillin molecule but with oxygen in place of sulphur (Howarth *et al.*, 1976) (Fig. 7).

Substances with β-lactamase inhibitory properties have also been found to be produced by *Streptomyces olivaceus, Streptomyces fulvoviridis* and other strains of *Streptomyces.* The structures of these substances, which again resemble the penicillin nucleus, are shown in Fig. 7. The olivanic acids MM 4550, MM 13902 and MM 17880 are not only very potent inhibitors of the R_{TEM} and *K. aerogenes* β-lactamases, but also have high antibacterial activity against a wide range of organisms and enhance the activity of β-lactamase-labile penicillins and cephalosporins against resistant strains of bacteria. Recently Okamura *et al.* (1978) have reported that a compound coded PS5 has *β*-lactamase inhibitory activity and acts synergistically with penicillins. The structure of PS5 is clearly related to the olivanic acids (Fig. 7).

It should be noted that although the antibiotic thienamycin (Fig. 7) appears to have a structure similar to the olivanic acids, it differs in the stereochemistry at carbon-6. In thienamycin the hydroxyethyl side chain projects down below the plane of the *β*-lactam ring and the 5,6 protons are *trans* to one another, while in the olivanic acids the hydroxyethyl projects above the *β*-lactam ring and the 5,6 protons are in the *cis* configuration. The olivanic acids also differ in a further respect in that they are sulphated and *N*-acetylated. These differences may explain why thienamycin has not been described as having *β*-lactamase inhibitory properties.

Macromolecular inhibitors of *β*-lactamase have been shown to be produced by *Streptomyces gedanensis* ATCC 4880 (Hata *et al.*, 1972) and *Streptomyces* sp. (Miyamura and Ochiai, 1974).

CLAVULANIC ACID

β-lactamase Inhibition and Antibacterial Synergy

Clavulanic acid has inhibitory activity against the *β*-lactamases of both gram-negative and gram-positive bacteria (Reading and Cole, 1977) (Table X). Unlike inhibitors such as BRL 1437, the inhibition is of a progressive type, very much lower I_{50} values being obtained when the enzyme is incubated with inhibitor for 15 min prior to adding the substrate. The enhancing effect of clavulanic acid on the antibacterial activity of ampicillin against a range of resistant bacteria is illustrated in Table XI. Lower concentrations of clavulanic acid are required for antibacterial synergy compared with the concentrations of cloxacillin and BRL 1437 previously described. As can be seen from Table XI clavulanic acid has broad-spectrum antibacterial activity but of a rather low order and insufficient to explain the enhanced activity seen when mixed with ampicillin. Clavulanic acid is not effective at improving the activity of ampicillin against a bacterium whose *β*-lactamase is poorly inhibited by clavulanic acid (Reading and Cole, 1977). Neu and Fu (1978) have also found a correlation between affinity of clavulanic acid for *β*-lactamases of Enterobacteriaceae and its potentiation of the antibacterial activity of various penicillins and cephalosporins.

The mechanism of action of clavulanic acid when acting as an antibacterial synergist is further illustrated in Fig. 8 from which it can be seen that the enhanced antibacterial activity of ampicillin plus clavulanic acid against *K. aerogenes* A is associated with the prevention of destruction of the ampicillin.

Clavulanic acid

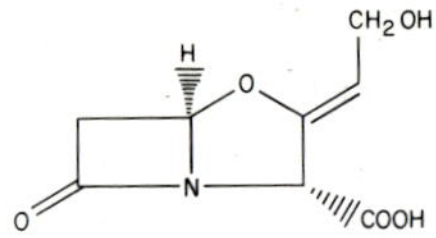

from *S. clavuligerus* ATCC 27064
Brown *et al.* 1976.
Howarth *et al.* 1976.
Reading and Cole, 1977
Brit. Pat. 1508 977.

Olivanic acids

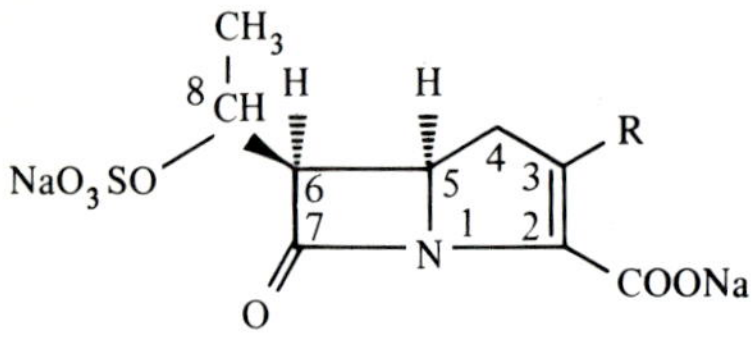

MM 4550 R =

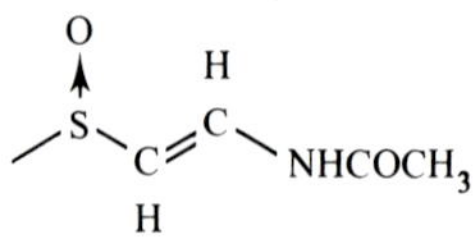

MM 13902 R =

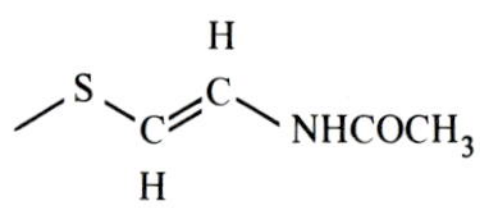

MM 17880 R =

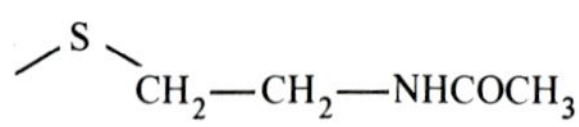

from *S. olivaceus* ATCC 21379
Brown *et al.* 1976.
Brown *et al.* 1977.
Corbett *et al.* 1977.
Brit. Pats. 1467 413, 1489 235 and 1483 142

MC 696-SY2 A — Structure as MM 4550 but stereochemistry not given.

from *S. fulvoviridis* ATCC 21954
Umezawa *et al.* 1973.
Maeda *et al.* 1977.

PS5

from *Streptomyces* spp.
Okamura *et al.* 1978.

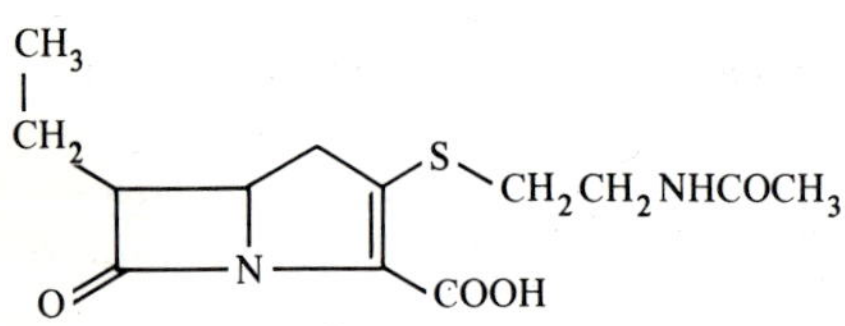

Thienamycin (structure given for comparison – not claimed to be ß-lactamase inhibitor)

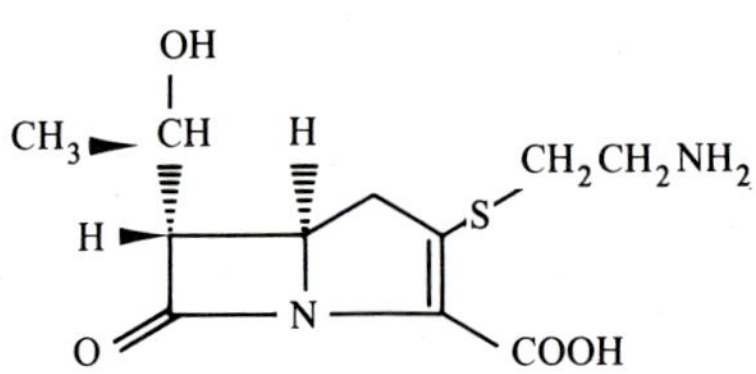

from *S. cattleya* NRRL 8057
U.S. Pat. 3950 357.
Johnston *et al.* 1978

Fig. 7 Clavulanic acid, olivanic acids and related structures—*ß*-lactamase inhibitors produced by *Streptomyces* spp.

TABLE X.

β-Lactamase inhibitory activity of clavulanic acid (BRL 14151). (From Beecham Pharmaceuticals, unpublished data.)

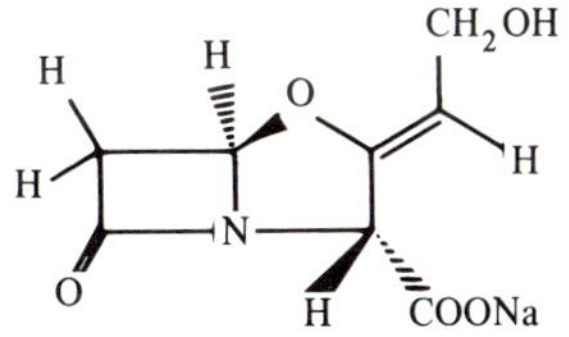

Source of β-lactamases	I_{50} values (μg ml^{-1}) Substrate* added immediately after inhibitor	Substrate* added 15 min. after inhibitor
E. coli K12 R TEM	0·56	0·08
E. coli JT 414	>>50	50
P. mirabilis C889	0·69	0·01
K. aerogenes A	0·11	0·01
Ent. cloacae NCTC 10005	>>50	c.50
Ps. aeruginosa A	>>50	>50
Staph. aureus MB9	0·84	0·02

* Substrate—benzylpenicillin 1 mg ml^{-1}.

TABLE XI.

Antibacterial activity of ampicillin against β-lactamase-producing bacteria in presence of sodium clavulanate. (From Reading and Cole, 1977.)

Organism	Minimum inhibitory concentrations* (μg ml^{-1})			
	Na-Clavulanate alone	Ampicillin alone	Ampicillin in presence of Na clavulanate 1 μg ml^{-1}	5 μg ml^{-1}
Staph. aureus (Russell)	15	500	0·8	0·02
K. aerogenes NCTC 418	31	250	0·4	0·1
P. mirabilis C889	62	>2 000	62	8
E. coli JT39 R+	31	>2 000	31	4
E. coli JT410 (chromosomal)	31	250	250	250

* Microtitre in tryptone soy broth. Inoculum 1/500 dilution of overnight broth culture.

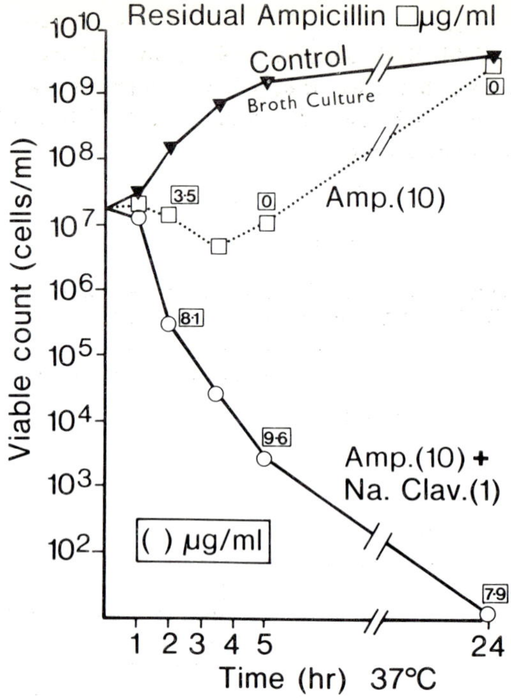

Fig. 8 Effect of ampicillin + Na clavulanate on growth of *Klebsiella aerogenes* A (from Beecham Pharmaceuticals, unpublished data).

Antibacterial synergy has been reported between clavulanic acid and benzylpenicillin, amoxycillin or cephalothin against *Bacteroides fragilis* and other species (Wise, 1977; Wüst and Wilkins, 1978), between clavulanic acid and cephalothin against *Klebsiella* strains (Jackson *et al.*, 1978), between clavulanic acid and benzylpenicillin or amoxycillin against various bacteria including *Staph. aureus, H. influenzae, E. coli, Klebsiella* and *B. fragilis* (Wise *et al.*, 1978) and between clavulanic acid and ticarcillin (Paisley, 1978). Reeves *et al.* (1978) have reported antibacterial synergism between clavulanic acid and amoxycillin or cephaloridine against a variety of gram-negative bacteria, and Sjöberg *et al.* (1978) have demonstrated much greater antibacterial synergy between clavulanic acid and ampicillin or carbenicillin against *H. influenzae* compared with that seen between mecillinam and these penicillins.

In a recent report by Ninane *et al.* (1978) the clinical effectiveness of a formulation of amoxycillin with clavulanic acid (BRL 25000, Augmentin®) was demonstrated in cases of chronic bronchitis involving a β-lactamase-producing strain of *Branhamella catarrhalis*. The results are summarized in Table XII, and the sensitivities of the isolated strains of *B. catarrhalis* to amoxycillin, clavulanic acid and BRL 25 000 are shown in Table XIII. Tests on the β-lactamase of one of these cultures of *B. catarrhalis* showed that it was readily inhibited by clavulanic acid, the I_{50} value being somewhat lower than that found for the TEM β-lactamase (C. Reading, personal communication).

TABLE XII.

Treatment of β-lactamase-producing bronchopulmonary infections with BRL 25 000.* (From Ninane *et al.*, 1978.)

	Coal miners with chronic bronchitis		
	Case 1	Case 2	Case 3
Previous treatment	Amp 3g/day oral for 7 days	Amoxy 1·5g/day 3 days	Amoxy 1·5g/day
Cultures present in transtracheal aspirate	*B. catarrhalis* (β-lactamase +ve)	*Str. pneumoniae* *H. influenzae* type b (β-lactamase −ve) *B. catarrhalis* (β-lactamase +ve)	*H. influenzae* type b *B. catarrhalis* (β-lactamase +ve)
Treated for 3 days with 2 tablets of BRL 25 000 three times a day			
Effect of treatment	Clinical improvement; sputum mucoid	Clinical improvement	Clinical improvement
Cultures present in transtracheal aspirate at 48 h after treatment	Sterile	Only *H. influenzae* type b (β-lactamase −ve)	Only *H. influenzae* type b (β-lactamase −ve)

* Each tablet contained 250 mg amoxycillin and 125 mg clavulanic acid.

Mechanism of Inhibition of β-lactamase

The interaction between clavulanic acid and the β-lactamase of *Staph. aureus* has been investigated by Reading and Hepburn (1979). Clavulanic acid was found to be a progressive inhibitor of this β-lactamase, the rate of inhibition increasing with increasing concentration of inhibitor. When the inhibitor is in molar excess over the enzyme, the reaction progresses in a first-order fashion with respect to inhibition.

The degree of initial inhibition of the β-lactamase is markedly reduced when

TABLE XIII.

Antibiotic sensitivity of β-lactamase-positive strains of *Branhamella catarrhalis* isolated from broncho-pulmonary infections. (From Ninane *et al.*, 1978.)

Drug	M.I.C. value (μg ml^{-1}) Case 1	Case 2	Case 3
Amoxycillin	50	25	25
Clavulanic acid	5	12·5	2·5
BRL 25000	0·05	<0·02	0·05

clavulanic acid is mixed with a high concentration of substrate (1 mg ml^{-1}) and the mixture added to the enzyme. The nature of the substrate influences the results as shown in Table XIV under the column headed "No preincubation". The type of substrate did not affect the magnitude of the I_{50} values when the inhibitor was allowed to react with the enzyme prior to adding the substrate. These results are explained by the initial phase of the inhibition of the enzyme by clavulanic acid being competitive with substrate. Substrates such as ampicillin have a lower affinity (higher K_m value) for the β-lactamase and thus have less interfering effect on the interaction between clavulanic acid and the enzyme.

The I_{50} values for the enzyme liberated by ultrasonics from the cells of several strains of *Staph. aureus* were in the region 0·1–0·12 μg ml^{-1} as shown in Table XIV,

TABLE XIV.

Clavulanic acid inhibition of β-lactamase liberated from the cells of *Staph. aureus* (Russell)—effect of substrate and preincubation time. (From Beecham Pharmaceuticals, unpublished data.)

Substrate (1 mg ml^{-1})	K_m (μM)	I_{50} values μg ml^{-1}: Preincubation (5 min. preincubation between inhibitor and enzyme before substrate added)	No preincubation (substrate and inhibitor mixed and added to enzyme)
Benzylpenicillin	14·5	0·12	43
Ampicillin	40·4	0·12	6
Amoxycillin	40·5	0·11	7

but were in the range 0·04–0·06 μg ml^{-1} for extracellular enzyme from the same strains. This difference could be explained by the effect of the attachment of the enzyme to wall fragments in the case of the ultrasonicated enzyme preparations.

The β-lactamase of *Staph. aureus* is not irreversibly inactivated by clavulanic acid. If benzylpenicillin is added to enzyme which has been completely inhibited by preincubation with clavulanic acid, activity very slowly returns. A similar effect is seen when clavulanic acid is removed by gel filtration.

The optimum pH for inhibition of the staphylococcal β-lactamase is pH 5·5–6·0 while the optimum for return of activity is less than pH 5·0. The initial binding of the enzyme to clavulanic acid is in the 1:1 molar ratio. The rate of destruction of clavulanic acid by the enzyme is very slow: enzyme which hydrolysed benzylpenicillin at 27 mg ml^{-1} min^{-1} hydrolysed clavulanic acid at 0·4 μg ml^{-1} h^{-1}.

The mechanism of inhibition of the R_{TEM} β-lactamase from *E. coli* is complicated and has been studied by Fisher *et al.* (1978), Charnas *et al.* (1978) and Reading and Farmer (in press). It has been found that two types of inhibited enzyme are

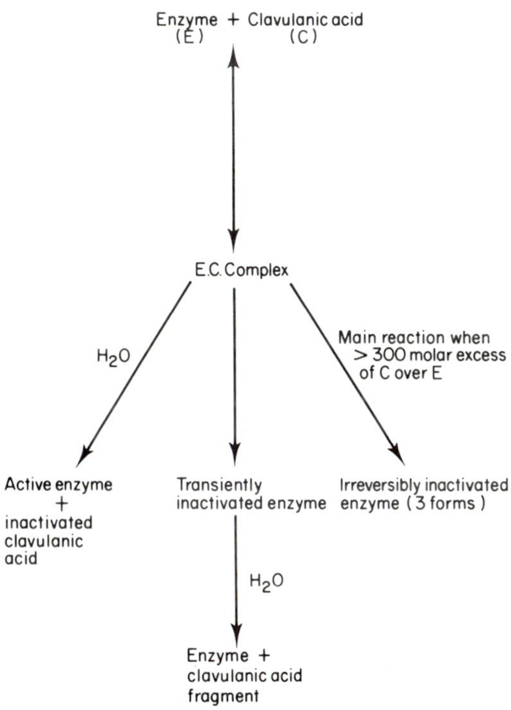

Fig. 9 Mechanism of inactivation of R_{TEM} β-lactamase by clavulanic acid (from Charnas *et al.*, 1978).

formed, irreversibly inactivated enzyme and transiently inactivated enzyme, the former predominating when clavulanic acid is in >300 molar excess over the enzyme. A scheme for the interaction is shown in Fig. 9 (Charnas *et al.*, 1978).

When using 1 μg ml^{-1} clavulanic acid the R_{TEM} β-lactamase is mainly in the irreversibly inhibited form even in the presence of substrate because of the high affinity between clavulanic acid and the enzyme. The R_{TEM} β-lactamase very slowly hydrolyses the clavulanic acid and Fisher *et al.* (1978) calculated that 115 molecules of clavulanic acid were needed per molecule of enzyme before the enzyme was completely inactivated. In a fully grown culture of *E. coli* JT4, an R-factor-containing strain, there was about 0·2μM β-lactamase which would require 4 μg ml^{-1} clavulanic acid to completely irreversibly inactivate it (Reading, unpublished data).

Neu and Fu (1978) have reported either competitive or non-competitive inhibition of β-lactamase when using enzymes from *Proteus, Pseudomonas* and *Klebsiella*.

Cherry *et al.* (1978) have recently described a derivative of clavulanic acid which has inhibitory activity against a wider range of β-lactamases than clavulanic acid as shown in Table XV. However, the activity against an important R-factor mediated β-lactamase is less than for clavulanic acid.

Various derivatives of clavulanic acid have been claimed in patents to have β-lactamase inhibitory activity, for example, deoxy clavulanic acid, carboxy esters,

TABLE XV.

Derivative of clavulanic acid with broad β-lactamase inhibitory activity. (From Cherry *et al.*, 1978.)

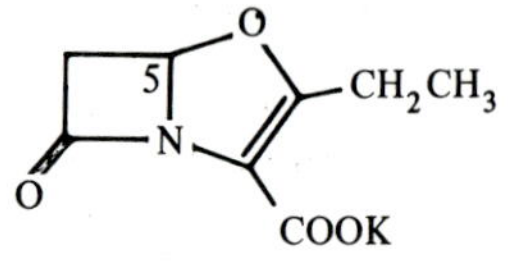

Compound 10 (5RS)

Source of β-lactamase	I_{50} values (μg ml^{-1})	
	Compound 10	Clavulanic acid
Staph. aureus PC1	0·02	8·2
Ent. cloacae P99	0·01	>25
RPI R factor	0·88	0·18
K. aerogenes K1	0·44	0·15

acylated derivatives, isoclavulanic acid derivatives, aminodeoxy derivatives, ethers and thioethers. Two synthetic analogues have also been described which have β-lactamase inhibitory activity (Bentley *et al.*, 1977; Hunt *et al.*, 1977).

CORRELATION BETWEEN β-LACTAMASE INHIBITION AND ANTIBACTERIAL SYNERGY

Generally, but not invariably, there is a good correlation between β-lactamase inhibitory activity and antibacterial synergy. Table XVI contains data obtained by O'Callaghan and Morris (1972) and shows that cloxacillin is a good inhibitor of the β-lactamase of *Ent. cloacae* and gives antibacterial synergy in combination with cephaloridine, whereas no synergy was seen with other organisms for which β-lactamases were poorly inhibited by cloxacillin. On the other hand, the correlation was not so obvious with α-naphthamido cephalosporanic acid as inhibitor, suggesting that other mechanisms may be involved.

Bach *et al.* (1967) found that good antibacterial synergy was only obtained with a competitive inhibitor when the K_m for the inhibitor was less than 0·1% of the K_m value for the labile antibiotic, i.e., the affinity of the inhibitor for the enzyme was over 1000 times the affinity of the substrate for the enzyme. This is illustrated in

TABLE XVI.

Correlation between β-lactamase inhibition and antibacterial synergy. (From O'Callaghan and Morris, 1972.)

Inhibitor	Source of β-lactamase	β-lactamase inhibition I_{50} (μM) (cephaloridine substrate at 100 μM)	Antibacterial synergy (fold reduction in MIC for cephaloridine when tested 1:1 with inhibitor)
Cloxacillin	*E. coli* R_{TEM}	16	No synergy
	Ent. cloacae P99	0·003	40 (Good synergy)*
	K. aerogenes K1	>100	No synergy
Nafcillin	*E. coli* R_{TEM}	0·02	4
	Ent. cloacae P99	0·03	8
	K. aerogenes K1	4	No synergy
α-Naphthamido cephalosporanic acid 443/1	*E. coli* R_{TEM}	5	8
	Ent. cloacae P99	0·3	No synergy
	K. aerogenes	80	No synergy

* MIC reduced from 2000 μg ml^{-1} to 50 μg ml^{-1} in presence of 50 μg ml^{-1} cloxacillin (MIC >1000).

Table XVII for the β-lactamase of *Shigella flexneri*. Farrar and Newsome (1973) determined K_i/K_m ratios and antibacterial activity for oxacillin and nafcillin as inhibitors with cephalothin as substrate when studying the β-lactamases of *Ent. cloacae, K. pneumoniae* and *Serratia marcescens*. Again antibacterial synergy was only seen when this ratio was in the region of 10^{-4} and not when it was 10^{-2}. The authors concluded that the observed synergy was due to inhibition of β-lactamase by one component and killing by the other. The concentrations required were higher than readily obtained in serum although they could be reached in urine.

Sabath (1968) stated four requirements for synergy by competitive inhibition of β-lactamase: (i) that β-lactamase must be an important factor in the organism's resistance; (ii) that the inhibitor must have very much greater affinity for the β-lactamase than the hydrolysable antibiotic to be protected (i.e. the K_i/K_m ratio must be very low); (iii) that the inhibitor must be stable to β-lactamase action; and (iv) that the inhibitor must have little or no antibacterial activity at the concentrations used.

Bobrowski *et al.* (1973) suggested a fifth requirement, namely that the inhibitor should be able to penetrate the cell wall at least as well as the labile antibiotic in view of the permeability barrier which exists to the site of action of cell bound

TABLE XVII.

Degree of β-lactamase inhibitory activity required for antibacterial synergy. (From Bach *et al.*, 1967.)

	Ampicillin K_m (μM)	Inhibitor K_i (μM)	K_i as a percentage of K_m	MIC for ampicillin (μg ml^{-1})	MIC for inhibitor (μg ml^{-1})	MIC (μg ml^{-1}) in broth for combination of ampicillin (set at 12·5 μg ml^{-1}) plus inhibitor
Shigella flexneri CDC 6533†	10	Dicloxacillin 0·0022	0·02	125	250	12·5 + 4–16*
		Methicillin 0·27	2·7	125	1 000	12·5 + 250–500
Aerobacter aerogenes (Yale)†	38	Dicloxacillin 4·7	12·0	125	1 000	12·5 + 500–1 000
		Methicillin 0·3	0·82	125	1 000	12·5 + 500–1 000

* Synergy seen in a mouse infection model.
† Similar results were obtained when benzylpenicillin was used instead of ampicillin.

β-lactamases. If intrinsic resistance to β-lactam antibiotics is present in a culture in addition to the ability to produce β-lactamase, antibacterial synergy with a β-lactamase inhibitor may be limited or not observed at all.

An indirect application of β-lactamase inhibition by cloxacillin was reported by Maddocks and May (1969) and May and Ingold (1971). They have shown that it is possible to inhibit the enterobacterial β-lactamase in sputum of bronchitics and thereby prevent the destruction of ampicillin and allow it to exert its antibacterial activity against the underlying causal organism *Haemophilus influenzae*.

MAMMALIAN β-LACTAMASE AND ITS INHIBITION

There is evidence to support the existence of mammalian β-lactamase although such an enzyme has not been isolated and characterized. Cole *et al.* (1973) demonstrated that for several penicillins there is a 30–50% breakdown to penicilloic acid in man. Experiments in animals (Kind *et al.*, 1968) suggest that the liver could be the site of inactivation. Inhibition of this apparent β-lactamase destruction might significantly increase the concentration of active antibiotic in the bloodstream. O'Callaghan (1978) has recently reported the inactivation of cephalosporins in human serum and has demonstrated the inhibition of the serum inactivation of nitrocefin (87/312) by another cephalosporin 10 485 (structure not specified).

CONCLUSION

Much progress has been made in developing satisfactory β-lactamase inhibitors. Several substances are currently undergoing further testing as antibacterial synergists, and clavulanic acid is being tested clinically. It remains to be seen to what extent β-lactamase inhibitors will be useful in treating infections involving β-lactamase-producing, resistant organisms but they have the important potential of extending the antibacterial spectrum of well-established antibacterial agents to include resistant organisms.

The most desirable properties which would be required for a β-lactamase inhibitor to be of use as a therapeutic adjunct are listed below:

(1) active against a wide range of clinically important β-lactamases;
(2) specific for β-lactamase;
(3) highly active in the presence of β-lactamase-labile antibiotics (substrates) either by competitive inhibition or rapid inactivation of the enzyme;
(4) active against cell-bound and exocellular forms of β-lactamase in growing bacterial cultures;
(5) stable to a wide range of β-lactamases;

(6) sufficiently active to be able to protect the antibacterial activity of the β-lactamase labile antibiotic and render resistant bacteria sensitive to concentrations of the labile antibiotic attainable in body fluids;
(7) low antibacterial activity and not an antibacterial antagonist;
(8) no interaction when mixed with β-lactamase-labile antibiotic;
(9) absorption and distribution characteristics similar to β-lactamase-labile antibiotic;
(10) low serum binding, minimal metabolism and low mammalian toxicity.

ACKNOWLEDGEMENTS

I should like to think my colleagues, Dr R. A. Edmondson and Mr C. Reading for β-lactamase inhibition data which I have quoted in various Tables; also Dr R. A. Edmondson for the isoelectric focusing results shown in Fig. 5, Miss Brenda Ridley for the K_m values in Table 14 and Mrs Pamela Hunter for the data in Fig. 8.

REFERENCES

Abbott, B. J. and Fukuda, D. S. (1975). Cephalosporin Acetylesterase *(Bacillus subtilis). In* "Methods in Enzymology **43** (Antibiotics)," (Ed. J. H. Hash), 731–734. Academic Press, New York and London.

Abraham, E. P. and Newton, G. G. F. (1956). A comparison of the action of penicillinase on benzylpenicillin and cephalosporin N and the competitive inhibition of penicillinase by cephalosporin C. *Biochemical Journal* **63,** 628–634.

Acred, P. and Sutherland, R. (1967). Antibacterial activities of combinations of ampicillin and cloxacillin. *Antimicrobial Agents and Chemotherapy—1966*, 53–58.

Bach, J. A., Buono, N., Chisholm, D., Price, K. E., Pursiano, T. A. and Gourevitch, A. (1967). In-vitro and in-vivo synergism of mixtures of penicillins. *Antimicrobial Agents and Chemotherapy—1966*, 328–336.

Behrens, O. K. and Garrison, L. (1950). Inhibitors for penicillinase. *Archives of Biochemistry* **27,** 94–98.

Bentley, P. H., Brooks, G., Gilpin, M. L. and Hunt, E. (1977). Total synthesis of clavulanic acid analogues via isomerisation of 7-oxo-4-oxa-1-azabicyclo-[3,2,0]hept-2-enes. *Journal of the Chemical Society Chemical Communications*, 905–906.

Benveniste, R. and Davies, J. (1971). Enzymatic acetylation of aminoglycoside antibiotics by *Escherichia coli* carrying an R-factor. *Biochemistry* **10,** 1787–1796.

Benveniste, R. and Davies, J. (1973). Mechanisms of antibiotic resistance in bacteria. *Annual Review Biochemistry* **42,** 471–506.

Bobrowski, M. M., Gebicka, K. and Borowski, J. (1973). Combined action of beta-lactam antibiotics against gram-negative bacilli. *Journal of Hygiene, Epidemiology, Microbiology and Immunology* **17,** 129–140.

Brown, A. G., Butterworth, D., Cole, M., Hanscomb, G., Hood, I. D., Reading, C. and Rolinson, G. N. (1976). Naturally occurring beta-lactamase inhibitors with antibacterial activity. *Journal of Antibiotics* **29,** 668–669.

Brown, A. G., Corbett, D. F., Eglington, A. J. and Howarth, T. T. (1977). Structures of olivanic acid derivatives MM 4550 and MM 13902; two new fused β-lactams isolated from *Streptomyces olivaceus. Journal of the Chemical Society Chemical Communications,* 523–525.

Charnas, R. L., Fisher, J. and Knowles, J. R. (1978). Chemical studies on the inactivation of *Escherichia coli* R_{TEM}beta-lactamase by clavulanic acid. *Biochemistry* **17,** 2185–2188.

Cherry, P. C., Newall, C. E. and Watson, N. S. (1978). Preparation of the 7-oxo-4-oxa-1-azabicyclo[3,2,0]hept-2-ene system and the reversible cleavage of its oxazoline ring. *Journal of the Chemical Society Chemical Communications,* 469–470.

Citri, N. and Pollock, M. R. (1966). The biochemistry and function of β-lactamase (penicillinase). *Advances in Enzymology* **28,** 237–323.

Cole, M. and Sutherland, R. (1966). The role of penicillin acylase in the resistance of gram-negative bacteria to penicillins. *Journal of General Microbiology* **42,** 345–356.

Cole, M., Elson, S. and Fullbrook, P. D. (1972). Inhibition of the beta-lactamases of *Escherichia coli* and *Klebsiella aerogenes* by semi-synthetic penicillins. *Biochemical Journal* **127,** 295–308.

Cole, M., Kenig, M. D. and Hewitt, V. A. (1973). Metabolism of penicillins to penicilloic acids and 6-aminopenicillanic acid in man and its significance in assessing penicillin absorption. *Antimicrobial Agents and Chemotherapy* **3,** 463–468.

Cole, M. (1979). Inhibition of β-lactamases. *In* "β-Lactamase" (Eds J. M. T. Hamilton-Miller and J. T. Smith), 205–289. Academic Press, New York and London.

Corbett, D. F., Eglington, A. J. and Howarth, T. T. (1977). Structure elucidation of MM 17880, a new fused β-lactam antibiotic isolated from *Streptomyces olivaceus*; a mild β-lactam degradation reaction. *J. Chemical Society Chemical Communications* 953–954.

Cronheim, G., Baird, M. E. and Dannenburg, W. N. (1949). Studies with penicillinase in presence of sulfonamides. *Archives of Biochemistry* **23,** 394–399.

Davies, J. E. and Rownd, R. (1972). Transmissible multiple drug resistance in Enterobacteriaceae. *Science (N.Y.)* **176,** 758–768.

Demain, A. L., Walton, R. B., Newkirk, J. F. and Miller, I. M. (1963). Microbial degradation of cephalosporin C. *Nature (London)* **199,** 909–910.

Farrar, W. E. and Newsome, J. K. (1973). Mechanism of synergistic effects of beta-lactam antibiotic combinations on gram-negative bacilli. *Antimicrobial Agents and Chemotherapy* **4,** 109–114.

Fisher, J., Charnas, R. L. and Knowles, J. R. (1978). Kinetic studies on the inactivation of *Escherichia coli* R_{TEM} beta-lactamase by clavulanic acid. *Biochemistry* **17,** 2180–2184.

Frère, J-M., Ghuysen, J-M., Vanderhaeghe, H., Adriaens, P., Degalaen, J. and De Graeve, J. (1976). Fate of thiazolidine ring during fragmentation of penicillin by exocellular DD-carboxypeptidase-transpeptidase of *Streptomyces* R61. *Nature (London)* **260,** 451–454.

Fu, K. P. and Neu, H. C. (1978). Kinetics of β-lactamase inhibition by HR-756, a new cephalosporin. Abstract A10 78th Annual Meeting of American Society for Microbiology, Las Vegas, May 1978.

Graber, H., Perenyi, T. and Arr, M. (1976). On human biotransformation of some penicillins. *International Journal of Clinical Pharmacology and Biopharmacy* **14,** 284–289.

Hass, M. J. and Dowding, J. E. (1975). Aminoglycoside-modifying enzymes. *In* "Methods in Enzymology **43** (Antibiotics)" (Ed. J. H. Hash), 611–628. Academic Press, New York and London.

Hamilton-Miller, J. M. T. (1963). Penicillinase from *Klebsiella aerogenes. Biochemical Journal* **87,** 209–214.

Hamilton-Miller, J. M. T. and Smith, J. T. (1964). Inhibition of penicillinases from gram-positive and gram-negative bacteria by substrate analogues. *Nature (London)* **201,** 999–1001.

Hammarström, S. and Strominger, J. L. (1976). Formation of 5,5-dimethyl-Δ^2-thiazoline-4-carboxylic acid during cleavage of penicillin G by D-alanine carboxypeptidase from *Bacillus stearothermophilus. Journal of Biological Chemistry* **251,** 7947–7949.

Hata, T., Omura, S., Iwai, Y., Ohno, H., Takeshima, H. and Yamaguchi, N. (1972). Studies on penicillinase inhibitors produced by microorganisms. *Journal of Antibiotics* **25,** 473–474.

Henry, R. J. and Housewright, R. D. (1947). Studies on penicillinase. II. Manometric method of assaying penicillinase and penicillin kinetics of the penicillin-penicillinase reaction, and the effects of inhibitors on penicillinase. *Journal of Biological Chemistry* **167,** 559–571.

Howarth, T. T., Brown, A. G. and King, T. J. (1976). Clavulanic acid, a novel beta-lactam isolated from *Streptomyces clavuligerus*; X-ray crystal structure analysis. *Journal of the Chemical Society Chemical Communications,* 266–267.

Hunt, E., Bentley, P. H., Brooks, G. and Gilpin, M. L. (1977). Total synthesis of beta-lactamase inhibitors related to clavulanic acid. *Journal of the Chemical Society Chemical Communications,* 906–907.

Hutter, S. and Welsch, M. (1948). Rôle d'une antipénicillinase dans les phénomènes attribués à la notalysine. *Comptes rendus des séances de la Société de biologie, Paris* **142,** 560–561.

Jackson, R. T., Harris, LeRoy F. and Alford, R. H. (1978). Sodium clavulanate potentiation of cephalosporin activity against clinical isolates of cephalothin-resistant *Klebsiella pneumoniae. Antimicrobial Agents and Chemotherapy* **14,** 118–125.

Jago, M., Migliacci, A. and Abraham, E. P. (1963). Production of a cephalosporinase by *Pseudomonas pyocyanea. Nature (London)* **199,** 375.

Johnson, K., Duez, C., Frère, J-M. and Ghuysen, J-M. (1975). *ß*-Lactamases (actinomycetes species). *In* "Methods in Enzymology **43** (Antibiotics)" (Ed. J. H. Hash), 687–698. Academic Press, New York and London.

Johnston, D. B. R., Schmitt, S. M., Buffard, F. A. and Christensen, B. G. (1978). The total synthesis of $\pm$ thienamycin. *Journal of the American Chemical Society* **100,** 313–315.

Kawaguchi, H. (1977). Recent progress in aminoglycoside antibiotics. *Japanese Journal of Antibiotics* **30** *Supplt,* S190-S200.

Kind, A. C., Beaty, H. N., Fenster, L. F. and Kirby, W. M. M. (1968). Inactivation of penicillins by the isolated rat liver. *Journal of Laboratory and Clinical Medicine* **71,** 728–735.

Kushner, D. J. and Breuil, C. (1977). Penicillinase (*ß*-lactamase) formation by blue-green algae. *Archives of Microbiology* **112,** 219–223.

Labia, R., Le Goffic, F., Faye, J-C. and Philippon, A. (1974). Deux céphalosporinases de *Pseudomonas aeruginosa. Biochimie* **56,** 1333–1337.

Maddocks, J. L. and May, J. R. (1969). Indirect pathogenicity of penicillase-producing entero-bacteria in chronic bronchial infections. *Lancet 1,* 793–795.

Maeda, K., Takahashi, S., Sezaki, M., Iinuma, K., Naganawa, H., Kondo, S., Ohno, M. and Umezawa, H. (1977). Isolation and structure of a *ß*-lactamase inhibitor from *Streptomyces. Journal of Antibiotics* **30,** 770–772.

May, J. R. and Ingold, A. (1971). Epiglottitis in adults. *British Medical Journal* **4,** 46.

Mahoney, D. F., Koppel, G. A. and Turner, J. R. (1976). Substrate inhibition of beta-lactamases, a method for predicting enzymatic stability of cephalosporins. *Antimicrobial Agents and Chemotherapy* **10,** 470–475.

Matthew, M., Harris, A. M., Marshall, M. J. and Ross, G. W. (1975). The use of analytical isoelectric focusing for detection and identification of *ß*-lactamases. *Journal of General Microbiology* **88,** 169–178.

Mehta, R. J. and Nash, C. H. (1978). β-Lactamase activity in yeast. *Journal of Antibiotics* **31,** 239–240.

Miyamura, S. and Ochiai, H. (1974). Inhibitors of beta-lactamases from gram-negative bacilli. Proc. 8th Int. Congress of Chemotherapy, Athens 1973. *In* "Progress in Chemotherapy" (Ed. G. K. Daikos), Vol I: 218–223 Hellenic Society for Chemotherapy, Athens.

Nayler, J. H. C., Long, A. A. W., Brown, D. M., Acred, P., Rolinson, G. N., Batchelor, F. R., Stevens, S. and Sutherland, R. (1962). Chemistry, toxicology, pharmacology and microbiology of a new acid-stable penicillin resistant to penicillinase (BRL 1621, cloxacillin). *Nature (London)* **195,** 1264–1267.

Neu, H. C. and Fu, K. P. (1978). The kinetics of β-lactamase inhibition by clavulanic acid. *Abstract A9, 78th Annual Meeting of American Society for Microbiology*, Las Vegas, May 1978.

Ninane, G., Joly, J. and Kraytman, M. (1978). Bronchopulmonary infection due to lactamase-producing *Branhamella catarrhalis* treated with amoxycillin/clavulanic acid. *Lancet* **ii,** 1978, 257.

O'Callaghan, C. H. (1978). Irreversible effects of serum proteins on β-lactam antibiotics. *Antimicrobial Agents and Chemotherapy* **13,** 628–633.

O'Callaghan, C. H. and Morris, A. (1972). Inhibition of beta-lactamases by beta-lactam antibiotics. *Antimicrobial Agents and Chemotherapy* **2,** 442–448.

O'Callaghan, C. H. and Muggleton, P. W. (1963). The formation of metabolites from cephalosporin compounds. *Biochemical Journal* **89,** 304–308.

Ogawara, H., Minagawa, T. and Nishizaki, H. (1978a). Property of the β-lactamase from *Streptomyces* E750-3. *Journal of Antibiotics* **31,** 923–925.

Ogawara, H., Horikawa, S., Shimada-Miyoshi, S. and Yasuzawa, K. (1978b). Production and property of β-lactamases in *Streptomyces*: comparison of the strains isolated newly and thirty years ago. *Antimicrobial Agents and Chemotherapy* **13,** 865–870.

Okamura, K., Hirata, S., Okumura, Y., Fukagawa, Y., Shimauchi, Y., Kouno, K., Ishikura, T. and Lein, J. (1978). PS-5, a new beta-lactam antibiotic from *Streptomyces*. *Journal of Antibiotics* **31,** 480–482.

Paisley, J. W. and Washington, J. A. (1978). Combined activity of clavulanic acid (BRL 14151) and ticarcillin on ticarcillin-resistant gram-negative bacilli. *Abstract A57, 78th Annual Meeting of American Society for Microbiology*, Las Vegas, May 1978.

Perlstein, D. and Liebmann, A. J. (1945). In-vitro protection of penicillin from inactivation by penicillinase. *Science (N.Y.)* **102,** 174–175.

Price, K. E., Pursiano, T. A., Defuria, M. D. and Wright, G. E. (1974). Activity of BB-K8 (Amikacin) against clinical isolates resistant to one or more aminoglycoside antibiotics. *Antimicrobial Agents and Chemotherapy* **5,** 143–152.

Reading, C. and Cole, M. (1977). Clavulanic acid: a beta-lactamase-inhibiting beta-lactam from *Streptomyces clavuligerus*. *Antimicrobial Agents and Chemotherapy* **11,** 852–857.

Reading, C. and Hepburn, P. (1979). The inhibition of staphylococcal β-lactamase by clavulanic acid. *Biochemical Journal* **179,** 67–76.

Reeves, D. S., Bywater, M. J. and Holt, H. A. (1978). Antibacterial synergism between beta-lactam antibiotics: results using clavulanic acid (BRL 14151) with amoxycillin carbenicillin or cephaloridine. *Infection* **6** *Supplt 1,* S9–S16.

Reid, R. D., Felton, L. C., Pittroff, M. A. (1946). Prolongation of penicillin activity with penicillinase-inhibiting compounds. *Proceedings of the Society for Experimental Biology and Medicine* **63,** 438–443.

Richmond, M. H. and Sykes, R. B. (1973). The β-lactamases of gram-negative bacteria and their possible physiological role. *In* "Advances in Microbial Physiology," Vol. 9 (Eds

A. H. Rose and D. W. Tempest) 31–88. Academic Press, London and New York.

Richmond, M. H. and Wotton, S. (1976). Comparative study of seven cephalosporins: susceptibility to β-lactamases and ability to penetrate the surface layers of *E. coli*. *Antimicrobial Agents and Chemotherapy* **10,** 219–222.

Rolinson, G. N., Stevens, S., Batchelor, F. R., Cameron-Wood, J. and Chain, E. B. (1960). Bacteriological studies on a new penicillin—BRL 1241 (Celbenin). *Lancet* **ii,** 564–567.

Rolinson, G. N. and Sutherland, R. (1973). Semisynthetic penicillin. *In* "Advances in Pharmacology and Chemotherapy," Vol. 11 (Eds. S. Garattini, A. Goldin, F. Hawking and I. J. Koplin), 151–220. Academic Press, London and New York.

Sabath, L. D. (1968). Synergy of antibacterial substances by apparently known mechanisms. *Antimicrobial Agents and Chemotherapy—1967*, 210–217.

Savidge, T. A. and Cole, M. (1975). Penicillin acylase (bacterial). *In* "Methods in Enzymology *43* (Antibiotics)" (Ed. J. H. Hash), 705–721. Academic Press, New York and London.

Shaw, W. V. (1975). Chloramphenicol acetyltransferase from chloramphenicol-resistant bacteria. *In* "Methods in Enzymology **43** (Antibiotics)" (Ed. J. H. Hash), 737–755. Academic Press, New York and London.

Shirley, R. L. and Moore, J. W. (1965). *Pseudomonas aeruginosa* urinary-tract infection. *New England Journal of Medicine* **273,** 283.

Sjöberg, B., Ekström, B., Forsgren, U., Magni, L. and Pring, B. G. (1978). Synergy of mecillinam and clavulanic acid with other beta-lactam antibiotics. *Infection* **6** *Suppl 1*, S17–S23.

Snow, G. A. (1962). Liver enzymes acting on methyl benzylpenicillinate. *Biochemical Journal* **82,** 6.

Sutherland, R. (1977). Synergic activities of penicillin combinations. *In Antibiotics and Antibiosis in Agriculture.* 3rd International Symposium, Sutton Bonnington, Loughborough. (Ed. M. Woodbine), 89–99. Butterworth, London.

Sutherland, R. and Batchelor, F. R. (1964). Synergistic activity of penicillins against penicillinase-producing gram-negative bacilli. *Nature (London)* **201,** 868–869.

Sykes, R. B. and Matthew, M. (1976). The β-lactamases of gram-negative bacteria and their role in resistance to β-lactam antibiotics. *Journal of Antimicrobial Chemotherapy* **2,** 115–157.

Tacking, R. (1955). Immunization experiments with penicillinase. *Acta Pathologica et Microbiologica Scandinavica* **36,** 61–65.

Tamura, T., Imae, Y. and Strominger, J. L. (1976). Purification to homogeneity and properties of two D-alanine carboxypeptidases I from *Escherichia coli*. *Journal of Biological Chemistry* **251,** 414–423.

Umezawa, H. (1970). Mechanisms of inactivation of aminoglycosidic antibiotics by enzymes of resistant organisms of clinical origin. *In* "Proceedings of the 6th International Congress of Chemotherapy. Progress in Antimicrobial and Anticancer Chemotherapy," Vol. II, 567–571. University of Tokyo Press, Tokyo.

Umezawa, H., Mitsuhashi, S., Hamada, M., Iyobe, S., Takahashi, S., Utahara, R., Osato, Y., Yamazaki, S., Ogawara, H. and Maeda, K. (1973). Two β-lactamase inhibitors produced by a *Streptomyces*. *Journal of Antibiotics* **26,** 51–54.

Vaczi, L. and Uri, J. (1954). Studies on the enzyme penicillinase. *Acta Microbiologica Academiae Scientiarum Hungaricae* **2,** 167–177.

Vining, L. C. (1975). Chloramphenicol hydrolase. *In* "Methods in Enzymology **43** (Antibiotics)" (Ed. J. H. Hash), 734–737. Academic Press, New York and London.

Wise, R. (1977). Clavulanic acid and susceptibility of *Bacteroides fragilis* to penicillin. *Lancet* **ii,** 145.

Wise, R., Andrews, J. M., Bedford, K. A. (1978). In-vitro study of clavulanic acid in combination with penicillin, amoxycillin and carbenicillin. *Antimicrobial Agents and Chemotherapy* **13**, 389–393.

Wüst, J. and Wilkins, T. D. (1978). Effect of clavulanic acid on anaerobic bacteria resistant to beta-lactam antibiotics. *Antimicrobial Agents and Chemotherapy* **13**, 130–133.

Yagisawa, M., Kondo, S., Takeuchi, T. and Umezawa, H. (1975). Aminoglycoside 6′-*N*-acetyltransferase of *Pseudomonas aeruginosa*: structural requirements of substrate. *Journal of Antibiotics* **28**, 486–489.

Zemelman, R. and Olivari, E. (1972). Carbenicillin as inhibitor of beta-lactamase from *Pseudomonas aeruginosa*. *Nature (New Biol.) (London)* **235**, 121–122.

DISCUSSION

Percival You did not mention Bacteroides. *B. fragilis* and related species have *ß*-lactamases, which are predominantly active against cephalosporins (but not cefoxitin) and are produced in varying amounts by different strains. These are also inhibited by clavulanic acid. In its presence, MICs of the most resistant strains (1000 μg ml^{-1} of ampicillin) are dramatically reduced (to 5 μg ml^{-1} or less) and of even the most sensitive strains to some extent. The latter presumably indicates the small part that low levels of constitutive enzyme play in determining susceptibility to *ß*-lactams. Similarly, I notice in one of your slides that *E. coli* and *Klebsiella* had MICs of 0·4 or 0·8 μg ml^{-1} of amoxycillin when combined with clavulanic acid. This is well below the sensitivity to amoxycillin of even the most susceptible strains in the absence of clavulanic acid and again reflects the small amounts of constitutive *ß*-lactamase activity possessed by all strains of these two species.

Cole The list of organisms for which synergy has been found has been extended beyond those on the slides and it certainly includes *Bacteroides*, as you say, and *H. influenzae*.

Kosmidis I have worked with Dr G. K. Daikos on the use of combination of amoxycillin and clavulanic acid in treatment of infections with ampicillin resistant bacteria. We were impressed by the in-vitro studies with this combination and we wanted to see if they work in clinical practice. We have therefore used tablets containing 250 mg amoxycillin + 125 mg clavulanic acid in 28 patients aged 18 to 76; 13 of these received one tablet three times a day and 15 received two tablets three times a day. All 28 infections were caused by ampicillin-resistant organisms, 22 urinary infections, two respiratory and four soft-tissue infections.

In 18 of these patients there were complicating factors which is why they had resistant organisms; in several, stones or malignancy were present and some of these cases had been unsuccessfully treated with other antibiotics. We carried out comprehensive toxicity studies in these patients before, during and after treatment. The results of the trial showed that in five cases of acute cystitis there was complete success. In some we did not have a satisfactory clinical result but 15 of a total of 22 urinary tract infections were cleared (Table I). We also obtained good results with five cases of infection outside the urinary tract including osteomyelitis.

There was a variety of infecting organisms including *Pseudomonas* and *Enterobacter* spp. and the results were satisfactory with all organisms (Table II). The cases that failed clinically were rather complex patients. One was a 65-year-old diabetic man with pyelocystitis caused by *E. coli* with multiple bladder papillomas. Previously he had been treated with cotrimoxazole and nalidixic acid and failed to respond. He was given the combination with initial improvement but recurrence of the symptoms and failure to eradicate the infecting organism. A 75-year-old man with prostate hypertrophy, residual bladder urine and hepatoma developed acute pyelonephritis with a *Citrobacter*. Previous therapy with cephapirin had failed. He was then treated with the combination with initial improvement

TABLE I.

Results of treatment with amoxycillin plus sodium clavulanate.

Diagnosis	No. patients	Clinical result				Bacterial result	
		Cure	Impr.*	Fail.	NA	Erad.	Pers.
Acute cystitis	5	5	—	—	—	5	—
Recurrent cystitis	3	2	—	1	—	1	2
Acute/recurrent cystitis on chronic active pyelonephritis	6	4	1	1	—	2	4
Acute pyelonephritis	2	1	—	1	—	2	—
Recurrent pyelonephritis	1	1	—	—	—	1	—
Asymptomatic chronic active pyelonephritis	4	—	—	—	4	3	1
Chronic urethritis	1	1	—	—	—	1	—
Osteomyelitis	1	—	1	—	—	—	1
Cellulitis	1	1	—	—	—	1	—
Carbuncle	1	1	—	—	—	1	—
Infected acne	1	1	—	—	—	1	—
Pneumonia	1	1	—	—	—	1	—
Exacerbated chronic bronchitis	1	1	—	—	—	1	—
Total	28	19	2	3	4	20	8

* Impr.—improvement, Fail.—failure, NA—not assessable, Erad.—eradication, Pers.—persistence.

TABLE II.

Results of treatment with amoxycillin plus sodium clavulanate according to the pathogen.

Species	No. patients	Clinical result: Cure	Impr.*	Fail.*	NA*	Bacteriological result: Erad.*	Pers.*
E. coli	3	2	—	1	—	2	1
C. freundii	2	1	—	1	—	2	—
K. pneumoniae	4	3	—	—	—	1	3
E. aerogenes	3	3	—	—	—	3	—
P. mirabilis	6	4	1	—	1	5	1
P. indole +	4	3	—	1	—	3	1
Providencia sp.	2	1	—	—	1	2	—
A. calcoaceticus var. *anitratus*	1	—	—	—	1	—	1
Staph. aureus	3	2	1	—	—	2	1
Total	28	19	2	3	4	20	8

*Impr.—improvement; Fail.—failure; NA—not assessable; Erad.—eradication; Pers.—persistence.

but deteriorated and the therapy had to be changed. A 65-year-old man with renal stones and acute pyelonephritis had had previous treatment with cotrimoxazole which had failed and when treated with the combination there was an initial clinical improvement but there was then relapse and the original pathogen was re-isolated. In all eight cases with bacteriological persistence there was one or more complicating factor. As far as side-effects are concerned there were some which could be attributed to amoxycillin; in two cases loose stools and in one a typical ampicillin rash which developed nine days after start of treatment. One case had a *Candida* infection on the first day. We did not have any other toxicity.

Kunin Early in my career I reviewed the text by Florey on penicillin. Deep in the text there is a statement that they had grown from the penicillin mould an agent which was a penicillinase inhibitor. They recommended that more work should be done on this subject. I did not note that in your history. We tried, unsuccessfully, to find that material. I believe for your own interest, Dr Cole, you may want to look back at that text. The early workers had the nub of the discovery back at that time. They did not, of course, characterize the substance except to mention that it was in the broth. I remember that very vividly because unfortunately I could not find it.

Cole I also have a recollection of seeing some such reference. I think you are referring to an antibiotic substance called notalysine. There is some French literature on this substance which seemed to be a β-lactamase-stable antibiotic but was later thought to be a penicillinase inhibitory substance produced by the *Penicillium* along with the penicillin. It might have an entirely different structure to penicillin.

Brumfitt There has been some discussion about toxicity of β-lactamase inhibitors in general and in particular clavulanic acid and liver toxicity. Did you investigate the enzymes or similar studies to see whether there was any such toxicity?

Kosmidis All the usual tests that are done during such studies were made, including alkaline phosphatase and other liver function tests before, during and after treatment and in only one case did we have a transitory rise of alkaline phosphatase. They were last done four days after stopping treatment.

Brumfitt I would say that was rather brief.

Mawer Has clavulanic acid any probenecid-like actions? Are the halflives in serum of the penicillins prolonged in the presence of clavulanic acid? Is any work being done on combinations of benzylpenicillin and clavulanic acid in patients with staphylococcal infections in combination with flucloxacillin and cloxacillin? There could be a good case for this combination.

Cole I don't know of any studies being done with benzylpenicillin. As for any probenecid-like action, I have not heard of any such report.

Smith Can Dr Cole give any evidence that the clavulanic acid is penicilloylating the enzyme when you get enzyme inhibition?

Cole Professor Knowles of Harvard has been studying the biochemical mechanisms of interaction between clavulanic acid and the R_{TEM} β-lactamase. He has just published two papers on this with his colleagues in the journal *Biochemistry*. The chemistry of the interaction is very complicated, particularly complicated for the TEM β-lactamase, because there are two types of inhibited enzyme—transiently inhibited enzyme and irreversibly inactivated enzyme.

When there is an excess of clavulanic molecules over enzyme molecules, e.g. over 300 molecules of clavulanic acid per molecule of enzyme, it is the irreversible inactivation route which predominates. If you have distinctly less, e.g. 50 molecules of clavulanic acid per molecule of R_{TEM} β-lactamase, then the transiently inhibited enzyme is formed. At a meeting in Strasbourg recently on enzyme inhibitors Knowles put forward the theory that only part of the clavulanic acid molecule, perhaps just a three-carbon fragment, is actually attached to the β-lactamase in such a way as to make it catalytically inactive.

Kass One can reasonably anticipate that every microorganism that makes a β-lactamase makes an inhibitor also. In theory one should be able to extract an inhibitor from the cell of any organism that makes a β-lactamase. Does the *Streptomyces* that makes the clavulanic acid also make a β-lactamase?

Cole There are many mechanisms by which enzymes which have been formed by the bacterial cell can disappear, and the production of a specific inhibitor is but one of many mechanisms. Another one is the thermal instability of the enzyme. Unfortunately the question you pose is very difficult to analyse because if, as one can postulate, the β-lactamase is going to be well inhibited you have got a problem to detect the enzyme. All I can say is that the clavulanic acids are very potent inhibitors of *Streptomyces* β-lactamase. But it is difficult to demonstrate production and inhibition of β-lactamase in the same organism unless the two activities are produced in distinct phases, for example early production of enzyme followed by later production of inhibitor. However, the enzyme inhibitors are usually produced early on in the growth of the organism.

Kass If one had a simple way of separating them we should then be able to test each β-lactamase from the organism that is causing whatever infection we are interested in. Sooner or later clavulanic acid will fail because there are organisms that have another way of getting round it and we will select for them. Either we develop synthetic analogues that are different enough so that this won't occur or else we must anticipate the selection of resistant organisms. From a therapeutic point of view it would be useful to have a simple way of finding the inhibitors so that we could cope with each strain as it came up.

Acar Does clavulanic acid bind to transpeptidases?

Cole Spratt published a paper on thienamycin and clavulanic acid and included their interaction with transpeptidase or penicillin-binding proteins. Clavulanic acid binds to the same protein as does mecillinam.

Antibiotic Synergism and Antagonism in Experimental Models of Infection

MERLE A. SANDE

University of Virginia School of Medicine,
Charlottesville, Virginia, USA.

INTRODUCTION

Since the work of Jawetz in the late 1940s, it has been clear that combining two antimicrobial agents may result in activity quite different from that of either drug alone (Jawetz *et al.*, 1951; Jawetz *et al.*, 1952). The resulting activity generally depends on the mechanism of action of the drugs. So-called bacteriostatic antibiotics such as the macrolides, chloramphenicol and the tetracyclines, work by reversibly inhibiting protein synthesis. They produce a therapeutic effect by stopping multiplication of the organisms and allowing host defences (phagocytic cells, antibodies, and complement) to eradicate the bacteria. Other drugs such as the penicillins, cephalosporins, vancomycin, and the aminoglycosides are bactericidal and are able to kill the bacteria by either producing a defect in the cell wall, or irreversibly binding to ribosomes. These agents require active metabolism and/or cell division of the bacteria in order to exert maximally their bactericidal activity. The addition of a bacteriostatic to a bactericidal drug, may, therefore, inhibit the bactericidal activity of these latter drugs, a phenomenon called antibiotic antagonism (White and White, 1964).

In other instances, combining two antibiotics may result in a more rapid or complete bactericidal effect than is produced by either drug alone. This has been called antibiotic synergism. A classic example is the combined action of penicillin and streptomycin against enterococcus (Jawetz and Gunnison, 1950). Neither drug is bactericidal against this species of *Streptococcus* alone, but the combination produced complete bacterial killing in broth. The action of penicillin on the cell wall increases the penetration of the aminoglycoside into the bacterium resulting in higher concentrations of the drug at the ribosome (Moellering and Weinberg, 1971).

The clinical relevance of these antibiotic interactions has been difficult to determine from clinical studies because of the complex nature of the factors that determine the outcome of bacterial infection. One might expect that in infections occurring in areas where the host's defence mechanisms are operative, a bacteriostatic antibiotic effect would provide adequate therapeutic intervention to tip the balance in the favour of the host. In such situations antagonistic combinations of antibiotics should theoretically not be detrimental as long as the combination is bacteriostatic against the infecting organism. On the other hand, in patients with impaired host defences or in infections located in areas where host defences are not maximally effective, bactericidal drugs or synergistic combinations might be expected to be of more critical importance and antagonistic antimicrobial combinations less effective.

The purpose of this paper is to present a series of experimental observations made in animals with various infections in which antimicrobial interactions are examined. The experimental data will be summarized and only the parts that are relevant to these aspects will be discussed.

ANTIMICROBIAL THERAPY OF INTRAPERITONEAL INFECTIONS IN NORMAL AND NEUTROPENIC MICE

Peritonitis is frequently a rapidly fatal infection that may be produced by the spillage of gastrointestinal contents from rupture of a viscus, or by surgical contamination. The bacterial aetiology of the infection is frequently mixed and includes group D streptococci, aerobic enteric bacilli, anaerobic streptococci, clostridia, and *Bacteroides fragilis*. The aerobic enteric bacilli may disseminate via the bloodstream from the infected site producing endotoxin shock and death. The anaerobes potentiate suppuration which results in tissue destruction and abscess formation. This condition has been reproducibly demonstrated in experimental animals (Onderdonk *et al.*, 1976).

The combination of gentamicin and chloramphenicol is frequently used to cover the spectrum of infecting organisms. However, in-vitro chloramphenicol will neutralize the bactericidal action of the gentamicin, and killing curves of the combination take on the bacteriostatic characteristics of chloramphenicol alone (White and White, 1964). A peritoneal infection was created in mice with the injection of 10^5 *Proteus mirabilis* and 5% hog gastric mucin (Sande and Overton, 1973). Mortality was 100% within 36 h. Therapy with gentamicin alone in a single dose cured 72% when started within 7 h following the infection. Chloramphenicol plus gentamicin was similarly effective and resulted in the survival of 47% of the infected animals ($P>0{\cdot}05$). When multiple dosages of drugs were administered 37% were cured with gentamicin alone and 61% with the combination. In these studies it appeared that host defences and polymorphonuclear leucocytes were mobilized in the peritoneal cavity and were able to eradicate the bacteria once multiplication had been stopped by the bacteriostatic effect. The bacteriostatic effect produced by the combination of drugs was not therapeutically inferior to the bactericidal effect of the gentamicin alone. Others have found similar results with gentamicin plus clindamycin in experimental intra-abdominal infection in rats (Weinstein *et al.*, 1975).

On the other hand, if the mice were first made neutropenic with total body irradiation, antibiotic antagonism became clinically significant (Sande and Overton, 1973). In these mice, only 10^2 organisms were required to produce a lethal intraperitoneal infection. Therapy with gentamicin alone with either single or multiple dosages resulted in survival of 93 and 89% of the animals, respectively, whereas therapy with the antagonistic combinations of chloramphenicol and gentamicin produced survival of only 40% and 39% ($P<0{\cdot}01$). These studies suggest that in animals with impaired host defences (a decrease in circulating polymorphonuclear leucocytes), the antagonistic combination was less effective than the single bactericidal drug alone. Clinical studies have suggested that synergistic antibiotic combinations have greater efficacy in the treatment of bacterial infections in neutropenic patients than single drugs or antagonistic combinations (Schimpff *et al.*, 1971; Klastersky *et al.*, 1972).

ANTIBIOTIC COMBINATIONS IN THE THERAPY OF EXPERIMENTAL BACTERIAL MENINGITIS

Clinical studies by Lepper and Dowling, and Mathies *et al.* have suggested that antagonistic antimicrobial combinations are less effective in the therapy of bacterial meningitis than a single bactericidal agent alone (Lepper and Dowling, 1951; Mathies *et al.*, 1967). These studies are frequently considered when selecting drugs for treatment of meningitis of unknown aetiology or meningitis caused by aerobic gram-negative bacilli. The aminoglycosides are generally recommended in these latter cases, but since inadequate CSF concentrations are achieved following parenteral administration intrathecal administration is necessary (Rahal *et al.*, 1974). Chloramphenicol, on the other hand, penetrates well into the CSF, but results of therapy with this drug alone have been inconsistent. The combination of gentamicin and chloramphenicol is therefore frequently used in an attempt to derive the beneficial contributions of each, i.e. the bactericidal effect of gentamicin and the enhanced CSF penetration of chloramphenicol. This approach as noted above is somewhat contradictory since in-vitro chloramphenicol inhibits the bactericidal effect of the gentamicin.

The purpose of the next study was to investigate the effect of adding chloramphenicol to gentamicin on bacterial killing in an experimental model of *Proteus mirabilis* meningitis (Strausbaugh and Sande, 1978). The organism used in these studies was the same as that used in the experiments above. Meningitis was produced by the intracisternal inoculation of 10^5 organisms. Eighteen hours later the animals were lethargic, febrile, and had purulent meningitis characterized by CSF pleocytosis, and an elevated protein. The animals were then suspended in a stereotaxic frame and treated with a constant i.v. infusion of either gentamicin alone, chloramphenicol alone, or the combination of gentamicin plus chloramphenicol for 8 h. Aliquots of CSF were removed at two-hour intervals for analysis of drug concentrations as well as quantification of viable bacteria. When gentamicin was given in dosages that achieved relatively high concentrations in the CSF, bacterial killing of up to 3 logs (from 10^5 to 10^2 bacteria per ml of CSF) occurred over the eight-hour treatment period. Chloramphenicol, on the other hand, as would be predicted from in-vitro time–kill curves, produced a bacteriostatic effect, while organisms from control animals increased by approximately one log (from 10^5 to 10^6 bacteria per ml of CSF). The addition of chloramphenicol to gentamicin completely eliminated the bactericidal effect of the gentamicin and produced a bacteriostatic effect identical to that seen with chloramphenicol alone. Thus, the addition of chloramphenicol to this therapeutic regimen eliminated the beneficial bactericidal effect achieved with the aminoglycoside.

Chloramphenicol, on the other hand, is bactericidal against some organisms such as *Haemophilus influenzae*, and its combination with other bactericidal drugs such as ampicillin does not produce antibiotic antagonism *in vitro*. The effect of the combination has also been studied *in vivo* in experimental *Haemophilus influenzae* meningitis (Bodine *et al*., 1977). Rabbits were infected with an intracisternal injection of 10^9 type b *H. influenzae* and treated as described above with a constant intravenous infusion of ampicillin alone, chloramphenicol alone or the combination. All three treatment regimens were equal and produced greater than 3 logs of bacterial killing (from 10^6 to 10^3 bacteria per ml of CSF) in the eight-hour treatment period. However, in experimental *Streptococcus pneumoniae* meningitis, chloramphenicol was bacteriostatic with no change in titre over the eight-hour treatment period. Ampicillin produced a drop of greater than 5 logs and the combination resulted in an intermediate effect; 4 logs of bacterial killing in 8 h. When 56 rabbits were treated for five days with one of the three regimens in doses that produced antibiotic serum levels that were similar to those considered therapeutic in man, the following was found: ampicillin-treated animals had a mortality rate of 26·3% and 11 out of 12 were sterile at the end of treatment; chloramphenicol treatment resulted in a 60% mortality and none of the animals surviving the five days of therapy had sterile CSF, while therapy with the combination produced a 44·4% mortality and 7 out of 10 rabbits had sterile CSF. When the dosage of chloramphenicol was increased to give serum levels of 50–100 μg ml^{-1} a bactericidal effect was produced (drop of 5·5 logs in 24 h) and the results of five-day treatment were similar to those of ampicillin alone. Thus, even though it may not always be possible to predict the final antimicrobial activity of such a combination of antibiotics, the results of time–kill curves *in vitro* seem to be predictive of their relative bactericidal activity and therapeutic efficacy in experimental meningitis.

Meningitis caused by *Listeria monocytogenes* is common especially in patients with compromised host resistance. Results of therapy have been discouraging and prompted a search for possible improvement with antibiotic combinations. Utilizing a modification of the meningitis model described above, the effectiveness of gentamicin plus penicillin, a combination which was found to be synergistic *in vitro*, was contrasted with penicillin alone, and penicillin plus rifampicin, a combination that was antagonistic *in vitro*. The rate of bacterial killing *in vivo* again reflected the effect *in vitro*. The reduction in bacterial titres with eight hours of continuous intravenous therapy were as follows: penicillin plus gentamicin $-2{\cdot}676 \pm 0{\cdot}655$, penicillin plus rifampicin $-1{\cdot}702 \pm 0{\cdot}495$, and penicillin alone $-1{\cdot}835 \pm 0{\cdot}555$ (Scheld and Sande, 1979. *Journal of Infection*).

These studies of *in vitro* and *in vivo* bacterial killing by antibiotics alone and in combination demonstrate that great variations exists between bactericidal activity of various therapeutic regimens. The single survival study suggests that the rate of bacterial killing might be important in determining success or failure of treatment. The few reported clinical studies support the concept that bactericidal drugs or combinations are superior in the treatment of meningitis to bacteriostatic or antagonistic antibiotic combinations (Lepper and Dowling, 1951; Mathies *et al.*, 1967).

COMBINATION ANTIMICROBIAL THERAPY OF EXPERIMENTAL BACTERIAL ENDOCARDITIS

The infection in bacterial endocarditis is located either on the endocardium or on the cardiac valve where the bacterial colonies are contained within a tight mesh of platelets and fibrin strands. The infected vegetation is remarkable for its sparsity of polymorphonuclear leucocytes or other phagocytic elements. This infection as it exists in the protected environment of the fibrin web should also be considered to be in an area of impaired host resistance. Clinical observations have consistently revealed that bacteriostatic antibiotics are ineffective in eradicating the infection in man.

In a series of studies we have demonstrated that the relative rate at which antibiotics alone or in combination kill bacteria in broth is predictive of the rate in which they eradicate the organisms from the cardiac vegetations *in vivo* in experimental endocarditis. A modification of the rabbit model of endocarditis first described by Freedman and colleagues was used in these experiments (Garrison and Freedman, 1970). The disease was produced by passing a polyethylene catheter into the carotid artery and across the aortic valve. The ensuing trauma to the endocardial surface stimulates the deposition of platelets and fibrin, which were then colonized by bacteria injected intravenously. Endocarditis can thus be produced with a wide variety of bacteria and fungi. The animals were treated with various antibiotics or combinations, sacrificed at given time periods, vegetations removed, quantitatively cultured, and the end-point of therapy recorded as number of viable bacteria remaining. In the first series of experiments, a strain of *Streptococcus sanguis* was used to produce the disease and nine days of penicillin therapy was required for sterilization of the vegetations and cure of the animals (Sande and Irvin, 1974). Discontinuation of therapy prior to cure resulted in relapse of the infection. The addition of an aminoglycoside, either gentamicin or streptomycin, to the penicillin therapy markedly increased the rate at which the bacteria were eradicated from the vegetation and achieved complete sterility in 3–4 days of continuous therapy. *In vitro* the combinations were more rapidly bactericidal than penicillin alone. A similar model of *Staphylococcus aureus* endocarditis was developed utilizing a penicillin-sensitive strain (Sande and Johnson, 1975). Penicillin alone required 7–9 days to produce complete sterility and cured the infection. Rifampicin was found to reduce the rate of bactericidal activity of the penicillin in broth and the combination was less effective in eradicating the bacteria from the cardiac vegetations in the experimental model. On the other hand, gentamicin was found to increase the rate of bactericidal activity produced by the penicillin in broth, and the combination was found to eradicate the organisms from the cardiac vegetations more rapidly than penicillin alone. These studies were confirmed, utilizing the same model with a penicillinase-producing *Staphylococcus aureus* (Sande and Courtney, 1976). Here the combination of gentamicin plus nafcillin was more rapidly effective than nafcillin alone.

As noted above, the enterococcus is particularly resistant to therapy with penicillin and the drug is usually not bactericidal *in vitro*. Penicillin is bactericidal when combined with streptomycin and this therapy has been effective in the disease in man (Mandell *et al.*, 1970). In the experimental model the combination was more effective than penicillin alone—mean bacterial titres were $10^{4 \cdot 8}$ colony-forming units per gram of vegetation in animals treated for 10 days with penicillin plus streptomycin, and $10^{6 \cdot 8}$ cfu g^{-1} of vegetation in animals treated with penicillin alone ($P<0 \cdot 05$) (Hook *et al.*, 1975). However, between 10% and 30%

of enterococcal strains isolated from patients with endocarditis are resistant to exceedingly high concentrations of streptomycin (>2000 μg ml^{-1}) (Moellering *et al.*, 1970). Synergism cannot be demonstrated *in vitro* with penicillin plus streptomycin against these strains since the aminoglycoside cannot bind to the ribosomes within the bacterial cell. Gentamicin does produce a bactericidal effect when combined with penicillin against these organisms. In the animal model of enterococcal endocarditis produced with a highly streptomycin resistant strain, the combination of penicillin plus streptomycin was no more effective than penicillin alone after 10 days of therapy. Vegetation titres were $10^{5.8}$ and $10^{6.6}$ cfu g^{-1} ($P > 0{\cdot}05$). Therapy with penicillin plus gentamicin was more effective than penicillin alone—$10^{5.0}$ versus $10^{6.6}$ cfu g^{-1} ($P < 0{\cdot}05$). Netilmicin, a new aminoglycoside, was also found to act synergistically with penicillin against the streptomycin resistant strains both *in vitro* and in experimental endocarditis, i.e. after 10 days of treatment vegetation titres from animals receiving penicillin plus netilmicin were $10^{4.7}$ compared with $10^{5.4}$ in penicillin-plus-gentamicin-treated rabbits (Korzeniowski *et al.*, 1978).

The above studies were carried out with *Str. faecalis*, the most prevalent of the enterococcal species. *Str. faecium* another strain of enterococcus which accounts for approximately 10% of clinical isolates was found to be more resistant to both penicillin and penicillin–aminoglycoside synergism. In fact, only penicillin plus gentamicin among all currently available aminoglycosides consistently produced a synergistic effect *in vitro*. In the animal model of endocarditis the penicillin–gentamicin combination produced mean vegetation titres of $10^{3.75}$ after 10 days of treatment compared to $10^{6.84}$ for the penicillin–netilmicin combination ($P < 0{\cdot}01$) and $10^{6.29}$ for penicillin alone ($P < 0{\cdot}01$). These observations again confirm the direct correlation of the rate of bacterial activity of antibiotic combinations in broth with their relative effectiveness *in vivo*.

Candida albicans has become a troublesome cause of endocarditis on prosthetic valves as well as on natural valves in narcotics addicts. Therapy with amphotericin is rarely successful. 5-Fluorocytosine, a fungistatic drug, has been shown to interact synergistically with amphotericin against some strains (Shadomy *et al.*, 1975). The addition of 5-fluorocytosine decreases the concentration of amphotericin required to inhibit the growth of *Candida albicans*. However, in our studies, it failed to decrease the concentration of amphotericin required to kill the fungus. In a rabbit model of *Candida albicans* endocarditis similar to that described above, amphotericin did eliminate the organism from the vegetations after six days of therapy (Sande *et al.*, 1977). 5-Fluorocytosine alone was fungistatic. The titres of organisms in the vegetations had not substantially changed after the six days of therapy. The addition of 5-fluorocytosine to the amphotericin therapy had no effect on the rate at which the amphotericin eradicated the fungus from the vegetations. Therefore, even though the combination produced an enhanced static effect over either drug alone, it did not demonstrate increased killing of the organism *in vitro* and had no detectable benefit over the single fungicidal drug in the experimental infection.

CONCLUSIONS

These experiments have examined the clinical significance of combination antimicrobial therapy in experimental infections. They have demonstrated that antibiotic antagonism was of little significance in an intraperitoneal infection when host defences were intact. The antagonism became relevant when animals were rendered neutropenic and their phagocytic capacity was reduced. In bacterial meningitis, polymorphonuclear leucocytes may not function optimally because of the inability of these phagocytic cells to trap the bacteria in the open spaces of the CSF. Several clinical studies suggest that bactericidal antibiotic activity may be important. Studies have demonstrated that the addition of chloramphenicol neutralizes the bactericidal effect of gentamicin both *in vitro* and in the experimental model of meningitis when the disease is caused by an aerobic gram-negative bacillus. Chloramphenicol was bactericidal against *H. influenzae in vitro* and produced no antagonism when combined with ampicillin in experimental *H. influenzae* meningitis. Bactericidal activity also is important in the therapy of bacterial endocarditis. This infection should be considered to occur in an area of impaired host resistance because of the inability of polymorphonuclear leucocytes to gain access to the bacterial colonies in the vegetation. The rate of bacterial killing produced by combinations in broth is predictive of the relative rate at which the organisms can be eradicated from cardiac vegetations *in vivo*. Synergistic combinations worked more rapidly and antagonistic combinations more slowly if at all. These studies demonstrate that the interaction of antibiotics may be particularly important in infections where maximal support from the host defence mechanisms is lacking.

REFERENCES

Bodine, J., Murray, T. and Sande, M. A. (1977). Combination therapy of experimental *Hemophilus influenzae* (HF) and *Streptococcus pneumoniae* (SP) meningitis. *Clinical Research* **27** A (Abstract).

Garrison, P. K. and Freedman, L. R. (1970). Experimental endocarditis. I. Staphylococcal endocarditis in rabbits resulting from placement of a polyethylene catheter in the right side of the heart. *Yale Journal of Biology and Medicine* **42,** 394–410.

Hook, E. W. III, Roberts, R. B. and Sande, M. A. (1975). Antimicrobial therapy of experimental enterococcal endocarditis. *Antimicrobial Agents and Chemotherapy* **8,** 564–570.

Jawetz, E. and Gunnison, M. A. (1950). The determination of sensitivity to penicillin and streptomycin of enterococci and streptococci of the viridans group. *Journal of Laboratory and Clinical Medicine* **35,** 488–496.

Jawetz, E., Gunnison, J. B., Bruff, J. B. and Coleman, V. R. (1952). Studies on antibiotic synergism and antagonism. Synergism among seven antibiotics against various bacteria *in vitro*. *Journal of Bacteriology* **64,** 29–39.

Jawetz, E., Gunnison, J. B., Speck, R. S. and Coleman, V. R. (1951). Studies on antibiotic synergism and antagonism. The interference of chloramphenicol with the action of penicillin. *Archives of Internal Medicine* **87,** 349–359.

Klastersky, J., Cappel, R., Daneau, D. (1972). Clinical significance of *in vitro* synergism between antibiotics in gram-negative infections. *Antimicrobial Agents and Chemotherapy* **2,** 470–475.

Korzeniowski, O. M., Wennersten, C., Moellering, R. C. Jr and Sande, M. A. (1978). Penicillin–netilmicin synergism against *Streptococcus faecalis*. *Antimicrobial Agents and Chemotherapy* **13,** 430–434.

Lepper, M. H. and Dowling, H. F. (1951). Treatment of pneumococcic meningitis with penicillin compared with penicillin plus aureomycin. [Studies including observations on an apparent antagonism between penicillin and aureomycin.] *Archives of Internal Medicine* **88,** 489–494.

Mandell, G. L., Kaye, D., Levison, M. E. and Hook, E. W. (1970). Enterococcal endocarditis. An analysis of 38 patients observed at the New York Hospital–Cornell Medical Center. *Archives of Internal Medicine* **125,** 258–264.

Mathies, A. W., Jr., Leedom, J. M., Ivler, D., Wehrle, P. F., Portnoy, B. (1967). Antibiotic antagonism in bacterial meningitis. *Antimicrobial Agents and Chemotherapy* 218–224.

Moellering, R. C. Jr, Korzeniowsky, O. M., Sande, M. A. and Wennersten, C. B. (1979). Species-specific resistance to antimicrobial synergism in *Str. faecium* and *Str. faecalis*. *Journal of Infectious Diseases* (in press).

Moellering, R. C. and Weinberg, A. N. (1971). Studies on antibiotic synergism against enterococci. II. Effect of various antibiotics on the uptake of C-labelled streptomycin by enterococci. *Journal of Clinical Investigation* **50,** 2580–2584.

Moellering, R. C., Wennersten, C., Medrek, T. and Weinberg, A. (1970). Prevalence of high-level resistance to aminoglycosides in clinical isolates of enterococci. *Antimicrobial Agents and Chemotherapy* **10,** 335–340.

Onderdonk, A. B., Bartlett, J. G., Louie, T., *et al.* (1976). Microbial synergy in experimental intra-abdominal abscess. *Infection and Immunity* **13,** 22–26.

Rahal, J. J., Hyams, P. J., Simberkoff, M. S., *et al.* (1974). Combined intrathecal and intramuscular gentamicin for gram-negative meningitis. *New England Journal of Medicine* **290,** 1394–1398.

Sande, M. A., Bowman, C. R. and Calderone, R. A. (1977). Experimental *Candida albicans* endocarditis. Characterization of the disease and response to therapy. *Infection and Immunity* **17,** 140–147.

Sande, M. A. and Courtney, K. B. (1976). Nafcillin–gentamicin synergism in experimental staphylococcal endocarditis. *Journal of Laboratory and Clinical Medicine* **88,** 118–124.

Sande, M. A. and Irvin, R. G. (1974). Penicillin–aminoglycoside synergy in experimental *Streptococcus viridans* endocarditis. *Journal of Infectious Diseases* **129,** 572–576.

Sande, M. A. and Johnson, M. L. (1975). Antimicrobial therapy of experimental endocarditis caused by *Staphylococcus aureus*. *Journal of Infectious Diseases* **131,** 367–375.

Sande, M. A. and Overton, J. W. (1973). In-vivo antagonism between gentamicin and chloramphenicol in neutropenic mice. *Journal of Infectious Diseases* **128,** 247–250.

Schimpff, S., Satterlee, W., Young, V. M. and Serpick, A. (1971). Empiric therapy with carbenicillin and gentamicin for febrile patients with cancer of granulocytopenia. *New England Journal of Medicine* **284,** 1061–1065.

Shadomy, S., Wagner, G., Espinel-Ingroff, A. and Davis, B. A. (1975). *In vitro* studies with combinations of 5-fluorocytosine plus amphotericin B. *Antimicrobial Agents and Chemotherapy* **8,** 117–121.

Strausbaugh, L. J. and Sande, M. A. (1978). Factors influencing the therapy of experimental *Proteus mirabilis* meningitis. *Journal of Infectious Diseases* **137,** 251–260.

Weinstein, W. M., Onderdonk, A. B. and Bartlett, J. G. (1975). Antimicrobial therapy of experimental intra-abdominal sepsis. *Journal of Infectious Diseases* **132,** 282–286.

White, J. R. and White, H. L. (1964). Streptomycinoid antibiotics: synergism by puromycin. *Science (N.Y.)* **146,** 772–773.

DISCUSSION

Percival You are now the saviour and hero of all the microbiologists because you have shown that what happens in the test-tube happens in the patient, or at least the infected animal!

Kass These are fine studies, and I am trying to put them into some clinical perspective.

First of all, if we go back to the early years of the successful treatment of bacterial endocarditis we are impressed by evidence that there were some cures with just a few days of treatment with penicillin, even in the doses that we used then. The doses got higher and the length of time was lengthened because experience accumulated to show that relapses were depressingly frequent without these approaches to treatment. That is why I am inherently concerned about reports that come out periodically that 10 days of oral therapy are sufficient. These reports are accurate enough, but I should prefer to see a large series because fundamentally our present treatment has been geared to the tail of the distribution curve of effect of dosage on recovery, and not to the majority of patients. Is there some realistic likelihood that there will be some few individuals in whom the treatment must be prolonged?

Secondly, we sometimes lose track of the literature on tetracycline, on sulphonamides. A few cures with these were always reported, but the numbers were small. We cannot be certain that all of these apparent cures occurred in patients with endocarditis, and there is no doubt of the greater effectiveness of bactericidal drugs. The point is that alternatives in an approach to treatment should include large numbers of patients before we can be sure of the efficacy of the approach in all patients. It will require collection of data on a large scale.

Sande There is a recent series (that I think is published from the Mayo Clinic) of 100 cases treated for two weeks with penicillin and streptomycin with no relapses. You could ask why did they switch to two weeks but it seems to me it is an ideal thing now to study. We have data *in vitro*, we have the data in animal models. It appears that we can rapidly eradicate the organism. It is cost effective if we can treat for two weeks rather than four.

Kass One of the relevant variables is that we are now using doses of penicillin that are several orders of magnitude larger than used previously. There is a reasonable possibility that we are getting more rapid sterilization of the lesion just because of that.

Brumfitt Regarding the *Streptococcus faecalis* endocarditis, why use benzylpenicillin and not ampicillin since ampicillin has been reported by a number of workers to be superior to any other β-lactam antibiotic in the therapy of *Str. faecalis* infections?

Sande Reports from Cornell examined very carefully ampicillin or penicillin versus *Str. faecalis*. In-vitro ampicillin was more active against *Str. faecalis* than penicillin alone. When they were compared in the rat model the cures were exactly the same. We use penicillin and not ampicillin probably because of tradition. Others have used ampicillin and I believe Dr Turck has cures with ampicillin alone. The rate of bactericidal activity could be about the same for both agents even although the MIC of ampicillin is lower.

Acar Have you studied different dosages of penicillin G to treat endocarditis with *Str. faecalis*? Have you any data concerning sensitivity *in vitro* to know if this has any relation to clinical results?

Sande We have not looked at different concentrations. We gave enough penicillin to produce serum concentrations of between 15 and 20 $\mu g\ ml^{-1}$ which is about what we achieved with 20 million units given intravenously over a 24-hour period.

Kunin I want to reiterate what Dr Kass said not only because it is rational but because I was house officer when the first failure occurred with short-course penicillin and streptomycin with endocarditis. I remember the case very well. When the series was going beautifully with a series of successes, one breakthrough occurred. I am very concerned about this issue because it seems to me that there is a temptation to try to separate prognostically staphylococcal bacteraemia due to a catheter as opposed to staphylococcal bacteraemia that may be due to endocarditis. These were thought to have different natural histories and therefore might be treated in a different fashion. It may be correct statistically to differentiate these episodes. I don't believe, however, it is relevant to use statistics since there are too many exceptions in severe infections. We must be very concerned to consider the fatal tail of a distribution curve. I see the temptation to ignore that tail on the basis of very small numbers of individuals studied.

I believe one has to be very careful about small series. One or two individuals might die because they don't fit into the distribution.

Williams It might be necessary to identify what is in that tail which makes those patients different. Are they host factors or merely that the organism is more resistant?

Kunin I don't know the answer, but suggest the following. Staphylococcal disease does not simply affect the heart valve but also many other tissues as well. There may be abscesses in multiple foci, depending on the host. He may have injured a bone or kidney at one time several years before and have a susceptible site. Mechanical failures are probably as important as immunologic disturbances. Most of us working in referral hospitals see that rare individual who comes in having been treated adequately for a staphylococcal infection for six weeks only to develop osteomyelitis or meningitis six months later. That is the tail as we see it. It is maybe a small number, but a therapeutic disaster.

Percival There are also dangers of over-treatment. Some suggest treating a highly sensitive *Str. viridans* endocarditis with 40 mega-units of benzylpenicillin a day through an in-dwelling catheter which they put into a big blood vessel. That has dangers.

Sande What I am looking at in the model is the rate of sterilization of the vegetation, but you are talking about something entirely different. You are probably talking about a standard abscess, perhaps in the heart or around the valve, that has relapsed. I certainly appreciate that difference and think it should be emphasized.

Kunin I appreciate that Dr Sande appreciates the difference. There is a problem with simplistic interpretation of animal data. I have to deal with house officers and infectious disease fellows, who literally treat according to animal data.

Percival What you are saying, then, is that because of the odd case which fails because there might, for example, be an abscess in the muscle by the valve, then you should treat all patients as if such a complication exists?

Kunin I am recommending that when one has a small series, even in humans, he may miss those few but important individuals. Therefore, I would rather err on the side of conservatism in prolonging therapy. The ethical question would be the misinterpretation of small series data. The problem is misinterpretation not by the author but by the people who conclude that this is great therapy, only to be disappointed when a few cases fail. This is Dr Kass' point.

Brumfitt There appears to be strong support for all patients with the streptococcal endocarditis to have a long course of treatment. However, some time ago I looked into the evidence that these vegetations did form quickly and caused emboli and I am not convinced that this is the case. At St Mary's there was a ward devoted to the study of bacterial endocarditis and after a course of treatment patients were very astute at knowing when they were relapsing and at returning to hospital rapidly for treatment. I have never seen the sort of disaster which Dr Kunin described. I do not think the evidence for short-term therapy is available and I don't know how we are going to get it but certainly we will not get it by giving everybody prolonged courses of treatment.

Jackson No one would argue with the treatment of staphylococcal disease. We are still collecting experience and there is very little evidence either from experimental animal models or from humans to suggest the short-term treatment is proper for staphylococcal endocarditis. I don't think it is.

Percival People sometimes get short-term treatment by default because 40%

of people with staphylococcal bacteraemia develop acute endocarditis as a secondary feature of that condition. When the blood culture is positive, I go to see all the patients and advise the clinicians to treat it as a case of endocarditis.

Kass Half the cases of staphylococcal endocarditis do not have a murmur. Experience leads many of us not to recommend short-term treatment for staphylococcal disease, although we have all seen cures with shorter courses. In the immunosuppressed patients, one would like to see a large series of patients to tell us whether static or cidal drugs are better in bacteraemia.

Sande In drug addicts it seems to be a different disease and the patients tend to do much better and are cured more rapidly.

Stuart-Harris We have given endocarditis an airing. Is there any other point that needs to be raised, for example about meningitis?

O'Grady Your animals with meningitis received five days' treatment, 100% were bacteriologically sterile but 40% of them died—what did they die of?

Sande They died early in the disease. If they survived to receive five days of high-dose therapy, cultures were sterile. There was an early mortality associated with the procedure. I did not make that clear.

I would question how effective chloramphenicol is for pneumococcal meningitis. This first came to be a strong recommendation for a penicillin-hypersensitive patient, following a series of articles in the *Maryland J. Med.* with the mortality rate 20%+. I would like to know how many of these strains have a difference between the MIC and the MBC and how many of them were really receiving bactericidal therapy. If you are not giving bactericidal therapy there may be a delayed response or failure.

Percival May I remind everyone that, for bacteraemia caused by gram-negative organisms, a recent review by McCabe (1975) showed that there was no difference between bactericidal and bacteriostatic agents in survival of two categories of patients: those who did not have an underlying disease and those with an ultimately fatal underlying disease. In the third category of those with a rapid fatal underlying disease, survival rates were greater when treatment was with bactericidal agents, but the numbers were far too small to be statistically significant. Therefore, in the one group where we might expect a difference there were not enough for assessment.

Kass Beware! We all know the pitfalls. We know very well of differences in the pathogenesis of disease in the animal model and in the human being. We know of the adverse effects of alcohol on the outcome of treatment of pneumococcal sepsis, and we know that mortality rates in hospitals that minister primarily to low-income patients are much higher than in more affluent populations.

Percival One question which I hope we will be able to answer during this meeting is "how often are combined courses of antimicrobials given? In what percentage of antimicrobial therapies in any particular countries are combinations used in comparison with single agents?"

Kass We can give you very exact figures on hospitals in the U.S.

REFERENCE

McCabe, W. R. (1975). Antibiotics and endotoxin shock. *Bulletin of the New York Academy of Medicine* **51,** 1084–1095.

The Toxicity of Antibiotic Combinations

GEORGE GEE JACKSON

University of Illinois, College of Medicine,
Chicago, Illinois, USA.

MEASUREMENT OF TOXICITY

In evaluating the toxicity of antibiotic combinations relative to one of the components, the incidence, severity and methods for the detection of toxic drug responses are important aspects of any comparison. The observed frequency of toxic reactions to a single or combination of antibiotics is a function of the nature of the toxicity and the system(s) available to detect their occurrence. The rates are lowest when recognition depends upon the development of objective clinical signs. Under these conditions the apparent rates vary according to the number of times and the diligence with which the signs are sought. Usually rates increase if the indicators of toxicity are looked for in a prospective fashion. The highest rates of drug toxicity are found when a simple sensitive test is available, such as the serum creatinine level or inner ear responses to a defined stimulus, which can reflect early even transient specific organ dysfunction that may be clinically inapparent.

To demonstrate an increased or decreased frequency of toxic reactions to a combination of antimicrobial drugs requires observations under conditions that are comparable (and usually simultaneous) with use of the single member drug. Only infrequently are such data available. Moreover, owing to the factors previously noted quantitative information about the overall toxicity of anti-infective agents used alone is poor. Thus, the observed frequency of reactions is a difficult standard of comparison except in direct comparative studies. Qualitative differences in the kind of toxic drug reactions offers another means by which the relative toxicity of an antibiotic combination can be evaluated. Such responses might also indicate a different mechanism of production of toxicity from that seen with the single antibiotic. In most cases of toxicity induced by combinations, however, the reaction is of the same type as that produced by the single drugs, except for the incidence or severity. Augmented severity can be simply the result of an additive effect, or the two drugs may be complementary in predisposing to toxicity. Conversely a decreased frequency or severity of toxicity can be achieved by using a lower dose of the toxic drug in a combination or possibly from a detoxifying action of the second antibiotic. The latter has been observed in animals, but is poorly documented if it occurs in man.

EXPRESSIONS OF ANTIBIOTIC TOXICITY AND OVERALL EFFECT OF COMBINATIONS

The use of anti-infective drugs as single agents has resulted in a wide variety of toxic reactions that can affect nearly every major tissue system in the body. Some of the more common categories and clinical expression of the reactions are given in Table I. Mostly the reactions are independent of the dose and the disease for which the drug was administered. The clinical manifestations do not permit recognition of subtle or perhaps even grossly additive or synergistic toxicity from drug combinations, or conversely a decrease in toxicity. If only death or life-threatening reactions to antibiotics are considered as the index, it can be implied from the remarkably low incidence of such reactions that there is no appreciable additive toxicity of such severity from combinations of antibiotics. In the surveys of fatal drug reactions by Jick and associates (Jick, 1974; Armstrong *et al.*, 1976), which included approximately 40 000 medical and surgical patients, the role of anti-infective drugs was almost nil. One knows from other data that approximately 30% of these patients received antimicrobial drugs and among those having major surgical procedures (4000–5000 in the surveys) treatment with antibiotic combinations would have been common. There were no antibiotic-related deaths. Thus, the overall rates of fatal reactions from antibiotics used singly or in combination is at most one in several thousand treated patients. At that low frequency of occurrence it must be concluded that death is not a toxic reaction that is appreciably changed by the use of antibiotic combinations.

TABLE I.

Major categories of antibiotic toxicity and some of its clinical manifestations.

Hypersensitivity	
	Eosinophilia — Rash, Contact dermatitis, Mucosal lesions — Fever — Anaphylaxis — Asthma — Lung infiltrates
Nephropathy	
	Cylindruria — Non-oliguric azotemia — Acute renal failure
	Proteinuria — Haematuria — Interstitial nephritis
	Diabetes insipidus (Vasopressin resistant)
	Fanconi's syndrome — Renal tubular acidosis
Gastrointestinal malfunction	
	Nausea and Vomiting — Colitis ($\pm$ pseudomembraneous)
	↑ Serum glutamic oxalic transaminase — Jaundice
	Malabsorption — Negative nitrogen balance — Hypovitaminosis B
	↓ Exocrine gland function
Ototoxicity and Neuropathology	
	Tinitis — Vertigo — High tone loss — Deafness
	Paresthesias — Neuromuscular blockade — Paralysis — Neuritis
	Convulsions — Confusion — Psychotoxicity
Haematological Abnormalities	
	Abnormal Coombs test — Haemolysis
	Granulocytopenia — Aplastic Anaemia
	Impaired coagulation
Electrolyte and Metabolic Disorders	
	Hypokalaemia — Lacticacidosis
Altered Host Defence Systems	
	PMNs ↓ Mobility ↑ Adherence ↓ Chemotaxis
	Lyphocytes, ↓ Mitogenic reactivity
	Antibody, ↓ Response
	Interferon, ↓ Response
Miscellaneous	
	Phlebitis — Cardiac enlargement
	Stained teeth (bone)
	Thyroiditis
	Direct Cytotoxicity — Foetal toxicity
	Photosensitivity

At the other end of the spectrum in the recognition of drug toxicity are measures that show extremely high rates, such as a small but significant increment in circulating eosinophils, enzymuria or a significant change in the daily excretion of granular casts in the urine. Using one of these as the index of drug toxicity yields

TABLE II.

Effect of concomitant drugs on rates of reactions to colistin. (From Koch-Weser *et al.*, 1970.)

Adjunct drug	Total utilizations		Renal reactions		Neural reactions	
Pressor agent	Yes	67	24%		6·0%	
	No	250	19%		7·6%	
Kanamycin or sulphonamide	Yes	66	24%		6·1%	
	No	251	19%		7·6%	
Cephalothin	Yes	78	33%	$P = < 0{\cdot}001$	11·5%	$P = < 0{\cdot}05$
	No	239	16%		5·9%	
Other aminoglycoside or β-lactam antibiotics	Yes	75	23%		9·3%	
	No	242	19%		6·6%	

reaction rates from single drugs as high as 40–80% with some antibiotics (Kluge and Wilkes, 1977; Giamarellou, 1977). The administration of combinations of antibiotics can accelerate or heighten the rate, but the differences observed and their clinical importance are usually of minor significance. It may be that such high rates offer the possibility to observe whether combinations can ameliorate the manifestations of a toxic component but none of the clinical studies documents this. Thus, using the two extremes in severity and frequency of drug reactions, there is no evidence to show that the use of antibiotic combinations either increases or decreases the overall toxicity of antimicrobial drugs to an appreciable extent.

SPECIFIC CLINICAL TOXICITY OF ANTIBIOTIC COMBINATIONS

Among non-fatal clinically important toxic reactions, a few have been recognised to occur in selected groups of patients with an increased frequency or severity from particular antibiotic combinations. Probably all three of the specificities noted—the kind of reaction, the patient characteristics, and the drugs involved—have importance in the creation of toxicity and the observed effect of the combination. Some of the reactions for which there is clinical documentation of an important difference between the use of a combination of antibiotics and the single members alone or in combination with other antibiotics are described below.

Nephrotoxicity

Renal reactions have occurred with colistin plus cephalothin significantly more often than with colistin alone (Table II). A combination of coli[illegible] ß-lactam antibiotic or a drug of a different class did not have suc[illegible] insufficiency has occurred more often with combinations of [illegible] either kanamycin, gentamicin or tobramycin than with the sam[illegible] combinations. This trend has been found in patients with acu[illegible] (Opitz *et al.*, 1971) and in those having cancer and/or bacteraemia (Klastersky *et al.*, 1975; Smith *et al.*, 1978).

Neurotoxicity

The inclusion of cephalothin in combination with colistin almost doubled the occurrence of neurologic reactions, which is statistically significant (Table II). Other ß-lactam antibiotics had a similar but less pronounced effect.

Hepatotoxicity

In combination, isoniazid and rifampicin increase the likelihood of hepatic injury to above that expected from either one alone, and perhaps greater than the sum of the two independently (Lal, 1972).

Electrolyte Disturbances

Hypokalaemia is produced with increased frequency by ticarcillin or carbinicillin when it is combined with cephalothin (Table III). The observed rate with the combination was almost double that with ticarcillin, but it is not statistically significant and can be corrected by the use of potassium supplements.

Allergic Reactions

The use of a penicillin and a cephalosporin together can produce skin rash in a greater proportion of patients than the sum of the number with rash from either one combined with an aminoglycoside (Table III). This is a statistically significant effect.

Role of Cephalothin

The prominence of cephalothin as a toxicity-potentiating member in several of the combinations can be noted in the foregoing reactions. This may be related specifically to cephalothin in those conditions involving failure of vital organ functions, but in the allergic reactions some of the effect can be assumed to be generic. It is possible that other cephalosporins will also produce a similar effect in most of the enhanced toxicity associated with cephalothin-containing combinations; however, only cephalothin has been used extensively enough to demonstrate the significance of the effect in clinical trials. The findings have considerable clinical importance because cephalothin, and other cephalosporins, are used mostly in antibiotic combinations. In part, the practice is followed because as a class cephalosporins are considered extremely safe, and there is little regard for the widely demonstrated potentiation of toxicity of other antibiotics when used as a combination with cephalothin. Later derivatives of cephalosporins should be studied both for their usefulness as therapeutic drugs when given alone and for their capacity to increase the toxicity of other antibiotics when used in combination.

SPECIFIC CLINICAL TOXICITY OF ANTIBIOTIC AND NON-ANTIBIOTIC COMBINATIONS

Antibiotic combinations in the context used here are considered to be two or more anti-infective agents. However, in the evaluation of the toxicity of antibiotics, it is important to note that they are often used in combination with non-antimicrobial drugs and that these combinations also can increase, exaggerate or alter toxic reactions to antibiotics. Among some commonly used drugs the potentiation of toxicity has been noted as follows.

Ototoxicity

Ethacrynic acid and aminoglycoside antibiotics mutually enhance the production of inner ear dysfunction that can be produced by either alone (Prazma, 1974).

Nephrotoxicity

Furosemide increases the renal damage produced by cephaloridine or cephalothin (Dodds and Foord, 1970).

Hepatotoxicity

Anaesthesia with halothane increases the occurrence of liver injury associated with rifampicin (Most and Markle, 1974).

Neural Toxicity

The administration of colistin or aminoglycoside antibiotics to persons taking muscle relaxants, or vice versa, increases the degree of neuromuscular blockade (Pittenger, 1970; Wright and McQuillen, 1971).

Electrolyte Disturbances

Corticosteroids enhance potassium depletion with Amphotericin B, sometimes resulting in cardiac enlargement (Chung and Koening, 1971), and perhaps increased nephrotoxicity (Kisch, 1978).

Rash

Allopurinol (and/or hyperuricaemia) increases the occurrence of rash from ampicillin (Boston Collaboration Study, 1972).

Other

The ingestion of alcohol can elicit a variety of adverse reactions of emotional or physiological nature in patients receiving any of several anti-infective medica-

TABLE III.

Adverse reactions to β-lactam antibiotics given as drug combinations to patients with cancer.

Regimen	N	Rash		Hypokalaemia	
I*					
Cephalothin + tobramycin		0/49	—	1/40	2%
Ticarcillin + tobramycin		2/54	4%	6/36	16%
Ticarcillin + cephalothin		5/50	10%	11/37	30%
II†					
Cephalothin + gentamicin	135		1%		17%
Carbenicillin (ticarcillin) + gentamicin	116		3%		22%‡
Carbenicillin (ticarcillin) + cephalothin	114		6%		25%‡

*I, From Klastersky, 1975.
†II, EORTC-JID, 1978.
‡Potassium given prophylactically.

tions; metronidazole, ethionamide and griseofulvin are among those that have been noted (Itel, 1978; Landsdown, 1967).

These various categorical reactions involving drug interactions with antimicrobials are only some examples of the development of clinical toxicity that have been observed as random occurrences in the treatment of patients. Undoubtedly, there are many more both recognized and unrecognized, but their detection is casual rather than systematic, and proof of specificity is often difficult. Owing to the widespread use of antimicrobial drugs, better definition of the extent and severity of these reactions would be desirable.

Examples of clinical conditions in which combinations of antibiotics or an antibiotic combined with other drugs have reduced drug toxicity are infrequent. Most of them are based on the application of antimicrobial synergy, usually of an aminoglycoside antibiotic in combination with penicillin or cephalosporin, which permits a decrease in the dose of one or both with resultant lessening of toxicity. A different mechanism is the relief of drug-induced reactions resulting from selective overgrowth or stimulation of pathogenic organisms that can be prevented by another antibiotic in the combination. An example might be the use of vancomycin for the prevention of clindamycin-induced colitis associated with *Clostridium difficile* (Lusk *et al.*, 1978). The reduction of drug toxicity in a pharmacologic sense, as a result of combining antibiotics at a dose equal to that when used alone, cannot be recognized in the controlled clinical trials.

INTERPRETATION OF TOXICITY FROM ANTIBIOTIC COMBINATIONS IN ANIMALS

The proper interpretation of the clinical findings observed with antibiotic combinations usually requires a better understanding of mechanisms and predisposing host factors than we have for most of the toxic reactions. Studies in animals have been designed to extend the controlled clinical observations and improve our knowledge about the cause and mediators of the increased or decreased toxicity. Unfortunately, in relation to antibiotic combinations, they have often failed to be definitive or applicable. This can be noted by the experiments with gentamicin and cephalothin in the production of nephrotoxic lesions in rats in which the effect tends to be opposite to that observed in man (Roos and Jackson, 1978; Luft, 1976; Dellinger, 1976). Similarly there is controversy about the clinical applicability of synergy and antagonism of antibiotic combinations which can often be demonstrated by the regulated conditions of animal experiments. The experience indicates that the drug reactions with combinations can be quite species- and/or disease-specific. It is necessary to use animal models to explore dose effects, time relations, comparison of related compounds and possible mechanisms of action. However, the most meaningful results must be obtained by careful evaluations from controlled clinical trials.

CONTROLLED CLINICAL TRIALS USING AN AMINOGLYCOSIDE PLUS CEPHALOTHIN

The most extensive controlled information pertains to the effect of cephalothin or another β-lactam antibiotic in the production of nephrotoxicity associated with aminoglycoside antibiotics. Although cephalothin alone or in combination with a penicillin infrequently causes nephrotoxicity it has been regularly observed to potentiate the transient and occasionally severe renal insufficiency caused by aminoglycosides and polymyxins. The results obtained in several controlled studies are given in Table IV. Using arbitrary but defined increments in the level of serum creatinine a significant augmentation of renal insufficiency was observed specifically with the combination of cephalothin and gentamicin or tobramycin. The effect is similar to the cephalothin associated increase in renal reactions with colistin (Table II). The majority of the investigations have been done in patients with cancer, and control groups given a single drug have not been included. However, the same trend has been observed among patients treated for gram-negative bacteraemia (Table IV, Group III). Therefore, cancer and its treatment are probably not the dominant factors in the occurrence of toxicity from the combination of antibiotics.

The frequency of nephrotoxicity varies considerably in the results of the different studies noted in Table IV; and also among the component subgroups of patients within the study centres. In the European trials, Groups I and II A, the doses of the antibiotics were generally uniform, plasma levels were not measured and the dose was adjusted only after nephrotoxicity was recognized to have occurred. All of these factors maximize the likelihood of differences in the results. On the regimens used, persons having good renal function would have developed only modest concentrations of aminoglycoside in the plasma with minimal drug accumulation and a low incidence of toxicity; whereas those patients with reduced kidney function would have progressive retention of the drug until functional toxicity occurred causing still greater retention until the nephrotoxicity became clinically apparent. The low frequency of toxicity when the aminoglycoside antibiotic (tobramycin) was used with a penicillin rather than cephalothin is most striking. In these protocols, such treatment served as the control group; however, it cannot be known with certainty that the penicillin did not have an effect, perhaps a beneficial one, either on a pharmacological basis or physiologically, due to improved anti-infective treatment for these patients with cancer.

In the American-based studies noted in Table IV, Groups II B and III, the blood concentration of aminoglycoside was monitored and adequate doses were

TABLE IV.

Effect of antibiotic combinations on the development of renal insufficiency.

Patient condition	Regimen % Reactions			Statistical significance
I SOLID TUMOUR	Gentamicin +carbenicillin +cephalothin		Carbenicillin +cephalothin	
	7/41 17%		1/40 3%	$P=0{\cdot}05$
LEUKAEMIA	Tobramycin +cephalothin	Tobramycin +ticarcillin	Ticarcillin +cephalothin	
Study No. 1	10/48 21%	3/53 6%	1/47 2%	$P=0{\cdot}05$
Study No. 2	22/135 16%	3/116 3%	6/114 5%	$P=0{\cdot}05$
II CANCER	Gentamicin +cephalothin	Gentamicin +carbenicillin (or ticarcillin)	Carbenicillin (or ticarcillin) +cephalothin	
A. Granulocytopaenia	16/35 12%	2/116 2%	4/114 4%	$P=0{\cdot}01$
B. ±Granulocytopaenia	— 25%	— 14%	— 6%	$P=$NS
III BACTERAEMIA	Gentamicin +cephalothin	Gentamicin +methicillin		
	8/23 35%	4/25 16%		$P=$NS
	Tobramycin +cephalothin	Tobramycin +methicillin		
	5/24 21%	1/26 4%		$P=$NS

I. Klastersky, J., 1978.
II A. EORTC, 1978.
II B. Bodey, G., 1978.
III. Smith, C. R., 1977.

I and II A: Regimen given without measurement of drug levels; dose adjusted after renal toxicity.
II B and III: Plasma drug level monitored and dose adjusted to give $\pm 10\,\mu g\,ml^{-1}$.

given to provide the desired level of $8\text{–}10\,\mu g\,ml^{-1}$. It is evident, with some exceptions, that when doses sufficient to maintain the blood level regardless of kidney function are given, the frequency of primary aminoglycoside nephrotoxicity is appreciably (and if it were in a comparative study, significantly) higher than with the European protocols. Of interest is the fact that the frequency of toxicity from the combination of gentamicin or tobramycin combined with cephalothin was not proportionately heightened by the maintained plasma levels of aminoglycoside, and the statistical significance of the differences is established with greater difficulty. These comparisons also lead to some different conclusions. In the EORTC investigations, the relation of toxicity to the patient's initial serum creatinine is noted, whereas the renal function is a negligible factor in the occurrence of toxicity when the serum concentration is kept constant. Nevertheless, from all of the data the trend is consistent that cephalothin specifically in combination with gentamicin or tobramycin increases the occurrence of antibiotic-induced renal insufficiency.

MECHANISMS BY WHICH ANTIBIOTIC COMBINATIONS ALTER TOXICITY

The mechanisms of the increased toxicity from cephalothin and gentamicin are not known. Pharmacokinetic data make it probable that the development of toxicity is related to more retention of the extremely stable aminoglycoside antibiotic (Schentag, 1978). In rats, where cephalothin has a beneficial effect on aminoglycoside-induced nephrotoxicity, one mechanism for the improvement is an accelerated or enhanced excretion of aminoglycoside (Roos and Jackson, 1977). Also, certain antibiotics cause vasomotor responses in the kidneys of rats and man that alter perfusion and the filtered drug load (Hollenberg, 1970). In view of the fact that the same combination of antibiotics can have an opposite effect on renal toxicity in rats and man, consideration must be given to the mechanisms whereby such results might be explained. A basis for these considerations is given in Table V. Improved drug elimination, possibly through the blockade of drug receptors or the elution of bound drug from tissue sites, could account for the relief of toxicity by cephalothin in rats. The adverse effect from cephalothin in man suggests that such a mechanism is inoperative and instead

TABLE V.

Nephrotoxicity or its prevention by antibiotic combinations.

Site	Mechanism(s)	Effect
Renal perfusion (urine)	Diuresis of drug	Accelerated excretion of toxic drug
	↓ Glomerular filtration ± Vasomotor shunts	Increased and/or prolonged retention
Tissue transport	Receptor blockade and/or Elution from tissues	Elimination of drug from tissues
	Facilitated unidirectional transport and/or intracellular trapping	Selective tissue deposition of drug
In situ (cellular)	Drug–drug or Drug–metabolite interactions	In-vivo detoxification or creation of toxic products

cephalothin might encourage the intracellular trapping of the stable aminoglycoside. Studies to date are compatible with such a thesis but they have not validated the logic. Another potential mechanism of the combination effect is through in-vivo drug interactions. When gentamicin and cephalothin are mixed *in vitro* there is a stoichiometric chemical reaction. The same reaction might occur in the kidney or other tissue if the local concentration of both drugs is high. The molecular derivatives of the interaction are microbiologically inactive and thus perhaps also not nephrotoxic in the rat. There is no evidence that any derivatives have enhanced toxicity, but if the reaction occurs at an intracellular locus it could alter the transport of the drug or other cell capabilities for handling the compounds with resultant tubular dysfunction.

HOST FACTORS IN NEPHROTOXICITY FROM AN AMINOGLYCOSIDE PLUS CEPHALOTHIN

The adverse effect of the combination of cephalothin and gentamicin in the causation of functional nephrotoxicity is strongly related to certain host characteristics. Two of these are noted in Fig. 1. It can be observed that the combination of aminoglycoside and cephalothin caused no nephrotoxicity among persons in whom the initial serum creatinine was <0·5 mg per 100 ml. Similarly it caused no

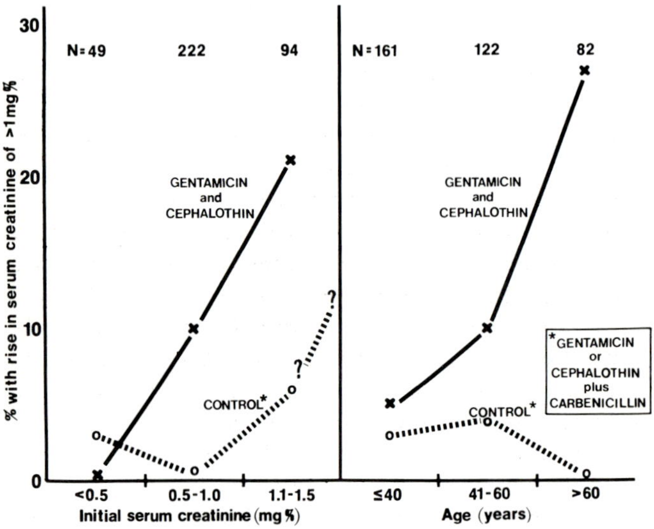

Fig. 1 Host factors in the development of nephrotoxicity from a combination of gentamicin and cephalothin or either one combined with carbenicillin. (Adapted from EROTC (Table 10), JID, 1978.)

enhanced toxicity compared to the control regimens in persons who were under 41 years of age. Marginally compensated states of renal function are stressed by the administration of gentamicin and more so by the combination regimen. As noted previously, if the plasma level of drug is not controlled, the frequency of nephrotoxicity rises with higher levels of initial serum creatinine. However, the difference between the individual drugs combined with carbenicillin (control group) and the test combination may occur only over a relatively narrow range of renal function. At more severe stages of renal insufficiency with an initial serum creatinine of >1·0 mg per 100 ml the rate of nephrotoxicity from uncontrolled dosage of aminoglycoside tends to catch up with that caused by the combination. When the ratio of nephrotoxicity in the test (gentamicin *plus* cephalothin) and the control (gentamicin *or* cephalothin with carbenicillin) groups is compared for different levels of initial serum creatinine (Fig. 1) the excess nephrotoxicity resulting from the combination decreases strikingly to an insignificant level when the initial creatinine is over 1·0 mg per 100 ml and as the overall incidence of nephrotoxicity increases with both regimens. This same host relation may also apply when the level of the aminoglycoside is controlled as was observed in the American-based investigations (Table IV). One reason for the smaller difference between the groups in persons with severely damaged kidneys might relate to Whelton's demonstration that severely diseased kidneys have different binding and extracting characteristics for aminoglycoside antibiotics than normal kidneys (Whelton, 1977). Although it is clear that the combination of gentamicin (or tobramycin) with cephalothin has an adverse effect related to renal function, the effect is most pronounced in a selected host population consisting of persons without renal failure, but having limited renal reserve. In persons with normal renal function or in those with advanced failure, the combination of antibiotic is not uniformly more toxic than the most toxic single component.

The effect of age on the development of nephrotoxicity from the combination of gentamicin and cephalothin is remarkably strong (Fig. 1). Over age 40 and especially after 60, there is a progressive increment in the excess nephrotoxicity from the combination above its occurrence from either component used with a penicillin. This effect of age is independent of the initial serum level of creatinine and is statistically significant when the data are corrected for it. Whether age has any other direct renal effect that increases susceptibility to the toxic effect of the combination is not known. The age factor could be related to the function of other organs, particularly the liver which in the case of cephalothin produces a 2-deacetylcephalothin derivative and excretes some of the drug. A similar effect of age and liver disease has been observed with INH toxicity either alone or in combination with rifamycin or alcohol (Kopanoff, 1978; Lals *et al.*, 1972). The data in Fig. 1 relate only to cancer patients who also have often been treated with anti-cancer drugs which might influence the results. Whether the striking importance of age *per se* in aggravating the adversity of the antibiotic combination also pertains in non-cancer patients can only be suspected until it is investigated in other patients.

One must conclude that antibiotic combinations in general do not fit a fixed pattern of causing increased or decreased toxicity. Often the increase in the breadth of spectrum or the ability to use lower doses of the most toxic drugs makes treatment with a combination of antibiotics attractive and effective. However, specific combinations of antibiotics are significantly more toxic than the components. The propensity to develop such toxic reactions is also determined by the clinical characteristics of the patients being treated. In future investigations, it will be important to separate further those variables.

REFERENCES

Armstrong, B., Denan, B., Jick, H. (1976). Fatal drug reactions in patients admitted to surgical services. *American Journal of Surgery* **132,** 643–645.

Bodey, G. (1978). Antimicrobial treatment of patients with cancer. Conference for evaluation of cephalothin and tobramycin in combination. Eli Lilly Co., Indianapolis, Indiana, U.S.A.

Boston Collaborative Drug Surveillance Program: Excess of ampicillin rashes with allopurinol or hyperuricemia. *New England Journal of Medicine* **286,** 1217. (1972).

Chung, D. K. and Koening, M. G. (1971). Reversible cardiac enlargement during treatment with amphotericin B and hydrocortisone. Report of three cases. *American Review of Respiratory Diseases* **103,** 831–841.

Dellinger, P., Murphy, T., Pinn, V., Barza, M. and Weinstein, L. (1976). Protective effect of cephalothin against gentamicin-induced nephrotoxicity in rats. *Antimicrobial Agents and Chemotherapy* **9,** 172–178.

Dood, M. G. and Foord, R. D. (1970). Enhancement by potent diuretics of renal tubular necrosis induced by cephaloridine. *British Journal of Pharmacology* **40,** 227–236.

EROTC. (1978). Three antibiotics regimens in the treatment of infection in febrile granulocytopenic patients with cancer. International Antimicrobial Therapy Project Group (European Organization for Research on Treatment of Cancer). *Journal of Infectious Diseases* **137,** 14–29.

Giamarellou, H., Petrikkos, G., Doudoulaki, P. and Daikos, G. K. (1977). Prospective comparative evaluation of gentamicin/gentamicin plus various cephalosporins with respect to nephrotoxicity in humans. Abstract No. 271, 10th International Congress of Chemotherapy, Zurich.

Hollenberg, N. K., Adams, D. F., Oken, D. E., Merrill, J. P. and Adams, D. F. (1970). Acute renal failure due to nephrotoxins: renal hemodynamics and angiographic studies in man. *New England Journal of Medicine* **282,** 1329–1334.

Itil, T. M., Holden, J. M. and Keskiner, A. (1968). Central effects of Methonidozol. *Psychiatric Research Report American Psychiatric Association* **24,** 148–165.

Jick, H. (1974). Drugs—Remarkably non-toxic. *New England Journal of Medicine* **291,** 824–828.

Kisch, A. L., Moydew, R. P. and Evan, A. P. (1978). Synergistic nephrotoxicity of Amphotericin B. and cortisone acetate in mice. *Journal of Infectious Diseases* **137,** 789–794.

Klastersky, J., Hensgens, C. and Debuscher, L. (1975). Empiric therapy for cancer patients:

comparative study of ticarcillin–tobramycin, ticarcillin–cephalothin, cephalothin–tobramycin. *Antimicrobial Agents and Chemotherapy* **7,** 640–645.
Kluge, R. M. and Wilkes, R. (1977). Reactions to antibiotics. *Journal of the American Medical Association* **237,** 1825.
Kock-Weser, J., Sidel, V. W., Federman, E. B., Kanarek, P., Finer, D. C. and Eaton, A. E. (1970). Adverse effects of sodium colistimethate: manifestations and specific reaction rates during 317 courses of therapy. *Annals of Internal Medicine* **72,** 857–868.
Kopanoff, D. E., Snider, D. E. and Caras, G. J. (1978). Isoniazid-related hepatitis. *American Review of Respiratory Diseases* **117,** 991–1001.
Lal, S., Singhal, S. N. and Burley, D. M. (1972). Effect of rifampicin and isoniazid on liver function. *British Medical Journal* **1,** 148–150.
Lansdown, F. S., Beran, M. and Litwak, T. (1967). Psychotoxic reaction during ethionomide therapy. *American Review of Respiratory Diseases* **95,** 1053–1055.
Luft, F. C., Patel, V., Yum, M. N. and Kleit, S. A. (1976). Nephrotoxicity of cephalosporin–gentamicin combinations in rats. *Antimicrobial Agents and Chemotherapy* **9,** 831–839.
Lusk, R. H., Fekety, R., Silva, J., Browne, R. A., Ringler, D. H. and Adams, J. D. (1978). Clindamycin induced enterocolitis in hamsters. *Journal of Infectious Diseases* **137,** 464–475.
Most, J. A. and Markle, G. B., IV. (1974). A nearly fatal hepatotoxic reaction to rifampicin after halothene anesthesia. *American Journal of Surgery* **127,** 593–595.
Opitz, A., Herrmann, I. and Herrath, D. (1971). Akute niereninsuffizienz nach gentamicin–cephalosporin kombinationstherapie. *Medizinischewelt* **11,** 434–438.
Pittenger, C. B., Eryasa, Y. and Adamson, R. (1970). Antibiotic induced paralysis. *Anesthesia and Analgesia* **49,** 487–501.
Prazma, J., Browder, J. P. and Fischer, N. D. (1974). Ethacrynic acid ototoxicity potentiation by kanamycin. *Annals Otology Rhinology and Laryngology* **83,** 111–118.
Roos, R. and Jackson, G. G. (1978). Protective effect of cephalothin on gentamicin nephrotoxicity; effect of cephalothin anion not sodium cation. Abstract No. 268. International Congress of Chemotherapy, Zurich.
Schentag, J. J., Lesezkay, G., Cumbo, T. J., Plaut, M. and Jusko, W. J. (1978). Accumulation pharmacokinetics of tobramycin. *Antimicrobial Agents and Chemotherapy* **13,** 34–40.
Smith, C. R., Baughman, K. L., Edwards, C. L., Rogers, J. F. and Lietmann, P. S. (1977). Controlled comparison of amikacin and gentamicin. *New England Journal of Medicine* **296,** 349–353.
Whelton, A., Carter, G. G., Bryant, H. H., Cody, T. S. and Walker, W. G. (1977). Tobramycin and gentamicin intrarenal kinetic comparisons therapeutic and toxicologic answers. Abstract 263. 10th International Congress of Chemotherapy, Zurich.
Wright, E. A. and McQuillen, M. P. (1971). Antibiotic induced neuromuscular blockade. *Annals of New York Academy of Sciences* **183,** 358–368.

DISCUSSION

Stuart-Harris On the first day Dr Percival made the point that one of the indications for combination therapy is that it might reduce toxicity.

Percival I would like to raise some questions about the use of aminoglycosides, first in combination with cephalosporins. There is nothing that a cephalosporin combined with an aminoglycoside can add in antimicrobial cover, which cannot be achieved with other agents, for example, clindamycin or, I suspect, erythromycin combined with an aminoglycoside. If metronidazole is used with the aminoglycoside, then a penicillin would have to be added to cover pneumococci or streptococci. Such combinations are, of course, mainly used for severe unknown or potentially mixed infections. The aminoglycoside–cephalosporin combination is potentially nephrotoxic and this is more likely to be a problem after surgery when there are often other causes of renal impairment than, for example, in leukaemics. Do we yet know if other complications like pseudomembranous enterocolitis occur more often after combinations than after single agents?

With aminoglycosides, it does not yet seem sufficiently to be appreciated that, in the presence of appreciable degrees of renal impairment, there is no way of achieving an adequate "peak" level without also creating a potentially toxic "trough" level. In a life-threatening infection, the risk of toxicity may have to be taken.

Jackson Regarding the problem of reduced toxicity or increased toxicity in relation to enterocolitis there are no data in man that say yes or no. In the animal model pretreatment with vancomycin will ameliorate or prevent the occurrence of the clindamycin-induced enterocolitis. You could call that a form of reduced toxicity from the combination. However, if the animal model reflects the correct pathogenesis of that disease, about which I have some reservations, then it is the prevention of an associated microbial disease and not a direct drug toxicity. Additionally, inhibition of DNA synthesis in colonic mucosa in culture has occurred when exposed to a number of different agents. The gut mucosa is a site of rapid DNA synthesis and has cells with short halflife. It could be affected by some antimicrobial drugs almost like bacteria. We still have to determine whether the enterotoxic colitis results from direct toxicity or from intoxication by a bacteriologic product. If the latter, an antibiotic that inhibits the organism producing the intoxicant would reduce toxicity.

I do not believe the relation of nephrotoxicity to the trough level of 2 μg aminoglycoside per ml is necessarily a toxic phenomenon; it is a reflection of inability to clear the drug. Renal insufficiency results in higher continuous levels and more nephrotoxicity, but I do not believe that justifies the conclusion that a trough level of $2\,\mu g\,ml^{-1}$ is in itself nephrotoxic. The level of $2\,\mu g\,ml^{-1}$ is the indicator of the non-clearance and therefore the subsequent toxicity rather than the cause of the toxicity. But I am not sure of that.

Percival What I meant about combinations to reduce toxicity is best illustrated by our recent experiences with endocarditis caused either by *Str. faecalis* or *Staph. aureus*. In three cases of each, we have successfully used 80 mg of gentamicin twice daily combined with ß-lactam antibiotics, because *in vitro* a total kill was achieved when concentrations of gentamicin considerably below its inhibitory levels were added to the ß-lactam. Also, we noticed that gentamicin alone was totally bactericidal at twice its M.I.C., which streptomycin was not. Two of the patients were allergic to penicillin and had also to be given "steroid cover", so there was anxiety about minimizing the β-lactam dosage. For *Str. faecalis*, the combination of gentamicin 80 mg twice daily with ampicillin 2 g i.v. six hourly was successful. Therefore we felt that the combinations were achieving a result which either agent alone might also have produced, but only at toxic dosage given for a relatively long period.

Jackson Yes, that is an important value of combination therapy but it is not reduced toxicity from the combination; rather it is the ability to use a reduced dosage of a toxic drug.

In discussing indicators of nephrotoxicity I left out the animal work which helps us to understand the mechanisms. The glycosidases are too sensitive as indicators but there are other enzymes such as alanine aminopeptidase which might be better. The various enzymes originate from different sites in the kidney. In addition there is some work on the leakiness of the glomeruli by measuring in agarose gel the size of the proteins in the urine. So there are techniques for us to examine not only the frequency but also the mechanisms and site of toxicity. At the moment they contribute no more than a general appreciation of the possible mechanisms and a future way to extend them.

Kass One recent piece of evidence on mechanisms is that gentamicin can be detected within the cells of the kidney tubule many days after the drug is no longer detectable in the urine. I wonder how many other drugs are in the situation in which storage in cells may occur for prolonged periods without being discarded by the cell. Clearly the toxicity of many of the drugs such as aminoglycosides is the main limitation to their more extended use at the higher dose level which sometimes we need to use. Enormous effort goes into remaking the molecule to increase activity. We know little about mechanisms of toxicity, so little effort goes into remaking the molecule to make it less toxic. The problem of testing toxicity in man is severely limiting.

Jackson Manipulations of the drug molecule to reduce toxicity have been of great interest. A disturbing fact is that the animal models are turning out to be somewhat non-predictive of toxicity in man. The animal models on which we have relied are not entirely satisfactory, for example netilmicin is absolutely non-toxic on the guinea-pig microphonics from the cochlea but in man it does not look like that is the case. The nephrotoxicity models of the rat with gentamicin and the cephalosporins have been absolutely inverted depending on what indices are chosen. We have all depended and must depend on animal screening before we get to the clinic but it is still true that the proof has to come from the clinical examination and it devolves on this group and others like it to make the kind of observations that permit us to recognize the early manifestations of toxicity.

Mawer Controlling concentration or monitoring concentration may protect against renal impairment in patients with renal disease but in our experience in Manchester it does not guarantee protection against ototoxicity which still remains a problem.

With regard to the point raised about serum creatinine concentration in the European series, it may be preferable to take serum creatinine concentration body-weight and age together to obtain an estimated creatinine clearance using the Danish nomogram rather than focusing attention on serum creatinine concentration.

A participant Dr Mawer's views on ototoxicity are eccentric in terms of the common consensus. Most experience has been the reciprocal of what has just been stated; the control of plasma levels will quite effectively control ototoxicity and, less effectively, control nephrotoxicity. Dr Percival was saying earlier that is what the trough level has been thought to be. I agree except that it is clearance of drug or failure of clearance which is related to nephrotoxicity. Most experience suggests that height of peak level is best related to ototoxicity and most of the consensus is in that direction at the moment.

Kunin It is possible that the drug receptors are different in the inner ear and kidney. Unfortunately I cannot cite the molecular formula presented as the chemical receptor of the ototoxic site, but there are data suggesting a very specific site whereas in the kidney it is much less clear. Some attempts have been made to look at why one aminoglycoside might be more toxic than another. We have looked at tissue binding of the drugs and under those circumstances we see in various tissues consistently across species lines that the most nephrotoxic agent is neomycin, streptomycin the least and that the other drugs are between. We have a new model which uses rabbit kidney because it is convenient to produce in the rabbit medulla. We combine ^{14}C-labelled gentamicin to the microsomes and then see which of the aminoglycosides will displace it in any kinetic patterns. The displacing agent fits exactly into the series of nephrotoxicity data already amassed. This need not necessarily be the answer but you can see a clear relationship and this seems to be a reasonable model for prediction.

Stuart-Harris This question of pseudomembranous colitis came up and I see Dr Larson is here. Would you like to comment at all on this?

Larson Pseudomembranous colitis (PMC) is an uncommon complication of antibiotic treatment, but cases do follow the use of antibiotics in combination. Recently, toxin-producing clostridia have been implicated as the cause of PMC (Larson *et al.*, 1977). A specific clostridial toxin can be identified in the faeces of patients by tissue culture neutralization test (Rifkin *et al.*, 1977) and toxin-producing *Clostridium difficile* are readily isolated (Bartlett *et al.*, 1978). This organism is very rarely isolated from normal subjects or those with other diseases, produces a toxin *in vitro* which is identical to that in PMC faeces, and induces enterocolitis when orally inoculated into susceptible hamsters (Larson *et al.*, 1978).

If PMC results from a bacterial infection, what role do antibiotics play in its induction? One possibility is that a resistant species overgrows the antibiotic suppressed normal flora. *Clostridium difficile* strains isolated from clindamycin-induced PMC have, in our experience, been clindamycin resistant. However, we have found strains from ampicillin-induced disease to be sensitive to that antibiotic, so that this explanation cannot apply to all cases of PMC. Pseudomembranous colitis was first described long prior to the antibiotic era and cases continue to be seen where antibiotics have not been administered. Further, we have not been able to establish that *C. difficile* is part of the faecal flora in healthy adults (Larson *et al.*, 1978).

Clindamycin induces an enterocolitis in hamsters resembling PMC in that both toxin and *C. difficile* are present. In spite of the fact that hamsters experience attack rates of 70–100% following either oral or intraperitoneal administration, *C. difficile* is not found in the faeces of animals prior to giving clindamycin. This attack rate drops to zero if animals are kept in a clean environment and given sterile diet and bedding, implying that infection with *C. difficile* is exogenous. If toxin-free suspensions of *C. difficile* are fed to untreated animals, no disease results. Apparently antibiotic treatment creates susceptibility to exogenous infection.

Besides clindamycin, lincomycin and ampicillin regularly induce *C. difficile* colitis in hamsters (four of four animals each). Penicillin induced disease in one of four, while tetracycline and metronidazole failed to induce disease. This parallels experience with human PMC in that clindamycin, lincomycin and ampicillin are the most commonly associated drugs. In 15 PMC patients who had received antibiotic combinations, these three drugs were also the most prevalent (Price and Davies, 1977), so that there are no data to suggest that commonly used combinations alter the disease incidence.

Lambert Vancomycin was one of the drugs for which colitis had been reported after parenteral administration and this is an interesting paradox. I have often before seen a drug pre-set the scene for development of infection and at the same time this may be the treatment for the established infection. From the way Dr Larson's work is developing we have to be very careful about our diagnosis and make sure we are treating established enterocolitis in the right way and not setting the scene for its development.

Larson I can only cite the recent paper by Dr Tedesco and his colleagues (Tedesco *et al.*, 1978) where 10 patients with established pseudomembranous colitis were treated with vancomycin. Nine received the drug orally and recovered; one was treated parenterally because she had had a colonic resection. This patient continued to excrete high levels of toxin in her faeces and eventually succumbed. No vancomycin could be detected in her stool. The presence of biologically active antibiotic in the stools may be important for the induction of pseudomembranous colitis as well as for its treatment.

REFERENCES

Bartlett, J. G., Chang, T. W., Gurwith, M., Gorbach, S. L. and Onderdonk, A. B. (1978). Antibiotic-associated pseudomembranous colitis due to toxin-producing clostridia. *New England Journal of Medicine* **298,** 531–534.

Larson, H. E., Parry, J. V., Price, A. B., Davies, D. R., Dobly, J. and Tyrrell, D. A. J. (1977). Undescribed toxin in pseudomembranous colitis. *British Medical Journal* **1,** 1246–1248.

Larson, H. E., Price, A. B., Honour, P. and Boriello, S. P. (1978). *Clostridium difficile* and the aetiology of pseumembranous colitis. *Lancet* **i,** 1063–1066.

Price, A. B. and Davies, D. R. (1977). Pseudomembranous colitis. *Journal of Clinical Pathology* **30,** 1–2.

Rifkin, G. D., Fekety, F. R., Silva, J., Jr and Sack, R. B. (1977). Antibiotic-induced colitis: implication of a toxin neutralized by *Clostridium sordelli* antitoxin. *Lancet* **ii,** 1103–1106.

Tedesco, F., Markham, P., Gurwith, M., Christie, D. and Bartlett, J. G. (1978). Oral vancomycin for antibiotic-associated pseudomembranous colitis. *Lancet* **ii,** 226.

Future Uses of Interactive Chemotherapy

H. P. LAMBERT

Department of Medicine,
St George's Hospital, London, UK.

FUTURE USES OF INTERACTIVE CHEMOTHERAPY

As every politician knows, prophecies are easy as long as one carefully eschews any attempt at dating them. I will share this cautious attitude in predicting the future of interactive chemotherapy, since some important advances seem to me as inevitable in their advent as they are uncertain in their timing.

Of the well-known uses of antimicrobial combinations, three can be described as interactive. These are the achievement of a superior, in the sense of more rapid and/or more complete, eradication of the infection, often by the action of antimicrobial synergy; the prevention of drug resistance; and the reduction of toxicity of individual components. Another common use of combined chemotherapy, the treatment of mixed infection at the same site, although at first seeming to possess no interactive element may, as we shall see, in fact involve important interactive components, while the other two uses of combined chemotherapy, broad "cover" for an uncertain microbial diagnosis and treatment of disparate infections in the same patient, do not involve interaction between the component agents (see Table I).

TABLE I.

Rationale of antimicrobial combinations.

Interactive	Non-interactive
Improve results by synergy	Initial treatment of serious infection, cause and/or drug susceptibility uncertain
Prevent resistance	Mixed infections (i.e. at same site)
Decrease toxicity	More than one infection (i.e. at different sites)

ERADICATION OF INFECTION

Mechanisms and examples of in-vitro and in-vivo synergy have been discussed in detail in this Symposium. The residual problems of clinical medicine for which such eradicative interactions will have their greatest value are precisely those infections which cause most difficulty now—infection in the immune-suppressed, whether by naturally occurring disease or more commonly, by therapeutic necessity, and those special examples of local immune suppression, the infected heart valve or vascular endothelium and infected prosthesis related to cardiac surgery or to cerebrospinal fluid shunts. Less dramatic but just as important is the hope that synergic combinations may, by early eradication of infection, prevent chronicity, relapse or latency with later breakdown in infections such as typhoid, brucellosis or melioidosis in which these features are especially troublesome.

The idea of combined treatment of this type involves two independent ideas, that of thoroughness of eradication and that of speed, and it is the latter which may be especially important in helping to achieve the second possible function of interactive chemotherapy, the prevention of resistance. Rapid eradication may be especially important in two different clinical problems. This aim has still not been achieved in the treatment of gonorrhoea and of some other sexually transmitted diseases. The other sphere in which rapid eradication may itself help to control the resistance problem is the treatment of carrier states. Munford *et al.* (1974) showed that a combination of minocycline and rifampicin was totally eradicative of the meningococcal carrier state, but one-third of the recipients suffered unwanted drug effects. Combined and non-toxic treatment for serious carrier problems, meningococcal, gonococcal, streptococcal and perhaps viral, is one of the advances we may look forward to.

Could eradicative combined chemotherapy have disadvantages?

First, chemotherapy of great speed and efficiency may lead to failure of immunity in those infections in which second attacks are normally rare or unknown. Secondly, could rapid eradication of virus infections for which subsequent latency is the norm open a Pandora's box which would have better stayed closed? What would be the population effects of the development of interactive antiviral chemotherapy leaving large numbers of adults without their latent infections with *Herpes simplex*, varicella-zoster, cytomegalovirus or EB virus? Long may such Frankensteins of chemotherapy be avoided!

PREVENTION OF RESISTANCE

We have already seen that one function of rapid eradicative chemotherapy is to avoid the resistance problem. In the longer term combination therapy is likely to remain of great importance in preventing the development of resistance in individual patients with particular types of pathogen or disease process, e.g. in tuberculosis, in antiviral, antifungal chemotherapy, in the treatment of urinary infections, and in certain forms of meningitis (especially in the neonate) and of course, in endocarditis. On the larger scale, however, it is hard to imagine any big impact by combination chemotherapy on the vast range of antimicrobial drug resistance in the population as a whole, simply because most such resistance does not arise in the context of individual treatment courses. Any benefit conceivable by massive use of combination chemotherapy for this purpose would be greatly outweighed by cumulative toxicity and expense. The path to decreased resistance is by restrictive rather than more complex prescribing policies.

PREVENTION OF TOXICITY

The third classic use of interactive chemotherapy also has an unpromising future. Since most adverse effects of antimicrobial agents are not critically dose dependent, antibiotic combinations are generally likely to be more toxic than single drug therapies. Some advances along the lines of the successful combination of low dose amphotericin B and flucytosine in fungal infections can, however, be anticipated (Utz *et al.*, 1975).

OTHER FORMS OF INTERACTIVE CHEMOTHERAPY: COMBINED THERAPY IN MIXED INFECTIONS

This form of combined chemotherapy is not normally considered as involving interaction between antimicrobial agents, since it is assumed that mixed infections, often of aerobes and anaerobes, should receive appropriate therapy for each component organism. Is it not illogical that we aim at a "kill-all" policy while commonly invoking the concept of bacterial synergy in this type of infection? If bacteria are acting synergically it must follow that inhibition of any of the component organisms would lead to effective control and that, if bacterial synergy could be reliably validated in clinical infections, we would need less rather than more combined chemotherapy. The truth is, of course, that our knowledge of the relationships of constituent organisms in mixed infections is still too scanty to provide us with really rational policies. But evidence of synergy is now emerging from experimental models, and in both directions. That is, of aerobic flora setting the biochemical scene for the establishment of anaerobic sepsis, and, more recently, of the reverse process. We have found (Hutchinson *et al.*, 1977), in experiments with metronidazole in a rabbit model of acute appendicitis, that, in addition to the expected decrease in the anaerobic flora, the aerobic flora showed a striking decrease in number and complexity. In later experiments, too, the number of gram-negative aerobes was no different in rabbits treated with erythromycin alone, active against the gram-positive aerobic cocci and against many anaerobes, and in those treated with erythromycin and gentamicin (unpublished experiments). Perhaps these findings are explained by the experiments of Ingham *et al.* (1977) on the inimical function of anaerobes on the capacity of leucocytes to deal with the aerobic flora.

INTERACTION OF ANTIMICROBIALS WITH DEFENCE MECHANISMS

The need for combined chemotherapy may thus be reduced by denying invading bacteria opportunities for synergic infection. A speculative look at the future of interactive therapy must also include possible advances, not between two or more antimicrobials, but between antimicrobials and other forms of adjuvant therapy, both specific and non-specific, since it is certain that advances will come from this direction. Again, mixed infections and abscesses provide a good example. Why does pus have to be drained? Why are abscesses difficult to sterilize? These ancient problems have long defied analysis, and it is refreshing to note renewed interest (Tally, 1978) in the physicochemical conditions in abscess cavities, and their effect on the activity of antimicrobial drugs. Improving the effect of single drugs by removing metabolic restriction of their activity is likely to improve results as much as the use of newer and better antibiotic combinations.

Another direction in which progress is already visible is the combination of chemotherapy with immunological adjuvant therapy. Several examples of combined action of an antiviral drug and specific antibody in the control of infection are available, such as the work of Cho and Feng (1977), showing enhanced protection in mouse infections with *Herpesvirus hominis* by the combined use of vidarabine and immune globulin. Synergic antiviral effects have also been demontrated against vaccinia virus in a tissue culture system by a combination of asparaginase and specific antiserum (Thiry and Cappel, 1975).

A complex experimental system which has revealed some important relationships is that developed by workers at NIH and Parke Davis on experimental *Pseudomonas* pneumonia in leucopenic dogs, of which the latest instalment was published last year by Kazmierowski *et al.* (1977). In an earlier, less severe, model of infection which was not accompanied by septicaemia, the best results were achieved with gentamicin together with granulocyte transfusions, although gentamicin with carbenicillin did almost as well. In the later models, in which the *Pseudomonas* culture was introduced into the distal airways with a fibroptic bronchoscope, *Pseudomonas* bacteraemia and pneumonia were regularly induced. In this system gentamicin had no observable effect. The combination of gentamicin with granulocyte infusions resulted in the survival of three out of eleven dogs, but those which died lived no longer on average than the controls. The administration of specific antibody (together with gentamicin) before inoculation of the infecting dose prolonged survival in proportion to the dose given but did not alter the pace at which blood and lung cultures became positive. The most effective therapy by far was provided by the combination of gentamicin, granulocyte transfusions and type-specific IgG antibody against the infecting serotype. With this combined approach six out of nine dogs were long-term survivors, compared with none out of 26 given gentamicin only, and the mean survival time of the three dogs which died was 6·0 days (2·9 days in controls).

Advances in therapy for the immune suppressed are surely likely to come from interactive therapies in this sense rather than by antimicrobial action alone.

PHARMACOKINETIC INTERACTIONS

Here prophecy could be virtually unbridled and I must confine myself to a single prediction. The word liposome was used by Bangham to denote a concentric closed-ring assemblage of phospholipid molecules, each representing an unbroken bimolecular sheet of lipid molecules which can be used to enclose a very large variety of agents and sonicated to form small monolamellar structures. This trapping of agents in liposomes determines their rate of clearance from the blood and their metabolic fate in the reticuloendothelial system (Gregoriadis, 1976). Substances entrapped in liposomes include a large number of enzymes, influenza virus haemaglutinin and neuraminidase, immunoglobulin, diphtheria toxoid, interferon inducers and some whole viruses. Some low molecular weight substances like benzylpenicillin and flucytosine do tend to diffuse out of liposomes, especially in the blood. These remarkable structures offer possibilities for the development of magic bullets of a laser-like accuracy which perhaps even Ehrlich himself could not have envisaged. Their possible applications in medicine range from neoplasia, inherited metabolic disorders, diabetes, and immunological adjuvants of unique power. And in microbial disease, one inevitably speculates whether here at last is a method of delivering agents at intracellular target sites with a greatly increased therapeutic ratio. In viral infections interferon induction can be improved by liposome entrapment and liposomes of defined composition can even be filled with viral particles, and, reverting to my theme of antimicrobial and immunological interaction, liposomes with antiviral antibodies can protect cells from virus infection. These findings in experimental systems are still a long way from application in man, but surely quite near are this year's reports of the use of antileishmania compounds in liposomes in the therapy of two forms of experimental leishmaniasis. The report by Alving *et al.* (1978) showed each of two liposome encapsulated antimonials 700 times as effective in this state as the corresponding drug in its normal form. The therapy of infections localized in the reticuloendothelial system which are often so hard to eradicate may yet benefit by such an approach.

EHRLICH ON DRUG COMBINATIONS

Although I have speculated on many possible and unfamiliar forms of combination chemotherapy, it remains true that the central ideas underlying the use of two or more antimicrobial drugs are those defined at the outset, that is, more effective eradication of the parasite, prevention of drug resistance, and reduction of toxicity. Although we have far to go in achieving these aims it would be wrong to suppose that the principles themselves are new. Ehrlich came to London in 1907 to deliver the Harben lectures at the Royal Institute of Public Health, entitled "Experimental Researches on Specific Therapeutics". In the last of them he uses the finding of resistance to different agents in trypanosomes to develop his concepts of specific points of therapeutic attack, and goes on to point out that ". . . the knowledge of the different points of attack is necessary, since it furnishes us with the possibility of fighting the disease by the combination of several chemotherapeutic agents". In the following pages he defines precisely the three main functions of interactive chemotherapy which we still recognize. These lectures were published in 1908, the year after they were delivered, so this meeting could be held both to recognize an anniversary and to continue the pursuit of the aims so well defined 70 years ago by the founder of modern chemotherapy.

REFERENCES

Alving, C. R., Steck, E. A., Chapman, W. L. Jr., Waits, V. B., Hendricks, L. D., Swartz, G. M. and Hanson, W. L. (1978). Therapy of leishmaniasis; superior efficacies of liposome-encapsulated drugs. *Proceedings of the National Academy of Sciences* **75,** 2959–2963.

Cho, C. T. and Feng, K. K. (1977). Interaction of adenine anabinoside and host defense factors in experimental infections due to *Herpesvirus homines*. *Journal of Infectious Diseases* **135,** 468–472.

Ehrlich, P. (1908). Experimental Researches on Specific Therapeutics, 91–95. H. K. Lewis, London.

Gregoriadis, G. (1976). The carrier potential of liposomes in biology and medicine. *New England Journal of Medicine* **295,** 704–709, 765–770.

Hutchinson, M., Lambert, H. P., Loughman, D. and Morgan, M. W. E. (1977). Metronidazole in experimental peritonitis. *In* "Metronidazole", Proceedings, Excerpta Medica, Montreal. 320–328.

Ingham, H. R., Sisson, P. R., Tharagonnet, D., Selkon, J. B. and Codd, A. A. (1977). Inhibition of phagocytosis *in vitro* by obligate anaerobes. *Lancet* **ii,** 1252–1254.

Kazmierowski, J. A., Reynolds, H. Y., Kauffman, J. C., Durbin, W. A., Graw, R. G. Jr and Devlin, H. B. (1977). Experimental pneumonia due to *Pseudomonas aeruginosa* in leukopenic dogs; prolongations of survival by combined treatment with passive antibody to *Pseudomonas* and granulocyte transfusions. *Journal of Infectious Diseases* **135,** 438–446.

Munford, R. S., de Vasconcelos, Z. J. S., Phillips, C. J., Gelli, D. S., Gorman, G. W., Risi, J. B. and Feldman, R. A. (1974). Eradication of carriage of *Neisseria* meningitis in families; a study in Brazil. *Journal of Infectious Diseases* **129,** 644–649.

Tally, F. P. (1978). Factors affecting antimicrobial agents in an anaerobic abscess. *Journal of Antimicrobial Chemotherapy* **4,** 299–302.

Thiry, L. and Cappel, R. (1975). Synergism between Antiviral Drugs in Clinical Use of Combinations of Antibiotics. 179–189. Hodder and Stoughton, London.

Utz, J. P., Garriques, I. L., Sande, M. A., Warner, J. F., Mandell, G. L., McGehee, R. F., Duma, R. J. and Shadomy, S. (1975). Therapy of cryptococcosis with a combination of flucytosine and amphotericin B. *Journal of Infectious Diseases* **132,** 368–373.

DISCUSSION

Brumfitt Synergy is something which we should all like to see but I wonder how often it really occurs. In the cotrimoxazole–trimethoprim mixture, the only clinical paper which shows synergy deals with the treatment of gonorrhoea. Are we looking for synergy in the right way? More important is the prevention of resistance, which is usually not a problem of a single episode of use but the multiple use of a drug often used incorrectly for inappropriate purposes on a large scale. Contrary to what one might suppose, giving streptomycin alone to a patient without active tuberculosis, rarely leads to that person excreting resistant tubercle bacilli. We must look very carefully at methods both in terms of the drugs we use and also how we use them in relation to preventing resistance, because all the trouble in failed chemotherapy stems from the development of resistance. The advantages of synergy although very attractive in theory are for selling drugs. It is much easier for a drug firm to say "Here is a combination which will kill more rapidly" than to say, "Here is a mixture which prevents resistance".

Brown I showed one slide where the polymyxin-resistant variant became progressively more sensitive to tetracycline. Have any studies been carried out on the spectrum of sensitivity of drug-resistant bacteria? For example, does resistance to gentamicin in *Ps. aeruginosa* (say by an exclusion mechanism) correlate with tetracycline sensitivity?

Smith The antibacterial activity of tetracyclines against *E. coli* in serum is enhanced and this is believed to be explained by the presence of complement affecting the envelope and thus affecting the activity of the drug. This is an example of the synergy, if you will, of the host bactericidal power with the antibiotic which could not exist in either alone.

A participant There are strains of gentamicin-resistant *Ps. aeruginosa* and many of these are also resistant to tetracycline.

Gilmore I will state briefly what antibiotic combinations I use as prophylaxis in high-risk patients undergoing gastrointestinal tract surgery and then ask the experts what I should be using with regard to both efficacy and the prevention of resistance. As you know, sepsis in surgery can have dire results, so in high-risk patients I use three doses of appropriate intravenous antibiotics. The first dose is given at the time of induction of anaesthesia and the second and third at 6 and 12 hours postoperatively. If during the operation unsuspected peritonitis is found then the antibiotic is given immediately intravenously.

In gastro-oesophageal surgery I use antibiotics in patients with carcinoma of the oesophagus, carcinoma of the stomach, pyloric stenosis or gastric ulcer only. In these patients I use a combination of flucloxacillin and gentamicin to protect against the staphylococci and the common gram-negative organisms.

In biliary surgery ampicillin and gentamicin are given to patients over 70 with a history of jaundice or previous biliary surgery or to anyone undergoing surgery within four weeks of acute cholecystitis.

In small bowel surgery antibiotics are only used in patients with obstruction ischaemia or Crohn's disease. In appendicectomy antibiotics are only used if the organ is gangrenous or perforated. For these patients and for all resections of the large intestine I use a combination of gentamicin and metronidazole. Gentamicin (120 mg) is given at the induction of anaesthesia with 500 mg of intravenous metronidazole. Gentamicin (80 mg) and 500 mg of metronidazole are given at 6 and 12 hourly intervals postoperatively. In elective colonic surgery I do not use oral preoperative antibiotics, but I consider mechanical preparation to be mandatory.

Jackson (?) One of our fundamental discussions has been the prevention of resistance by the use of combinations. In the prevention of resistant mutants combinations have been very effective we believe, as in tuberculosis, but it appears to be almost of no importance in most infections. The emergence of resistance due to plasmid transfer has become a difficulty, and combinations of antibiotics as a general rule are not very effective—they just build the size of the plasmid and the genes that are being carried. We do not have an effective way in terms of combinations for preventing that form of resistance. We must critically ask even in tuberculosis whether or not this repeatedly stated use for preventing the emergence of resistance is actually valid or not; we may be building more complex resistance into the ecology. There is also the third mechanism Dr Brown has put before us. There are a few glimpses of reciprocal changes of resistance to one agent and sensitivity to another, e.g. with staphylococcal and bacitracin versus tetracycline. These effects may be seen in epidemiologic and ecologic studies of clinical material. Usually they cannot be predicted from the laboratory and have to be seen after-the-fact to find the lessons for the future. In these three categories of prevention of resistance the mutational type is probably not of much importance; we fail in the prevention of resistance when it is plasmid-borne and we need to find more of the resistant–sensitive relationships of the reverse kind.

Index

Abdominal surgery, 6
Absorption, inteference with, 36, 37
Allergic reactions, 155
Aminoglycoside–inactivating enzymes, 101
  inhibition of, 102
Aminoglycosides
  and cephalosporins, 18
  and cephalothin, 159
  and penicillins, 18
    and nephrotoxicity, 162
Animal models of infection, 14
Antagonism
  between chloramphenicol and penicillins, 25
  clinical demonstration of, 28
Antibiotic antagonism in mice, 139
Antibiotic combinations, toxicity of, 151
Antibiotic–drug interactions, direct, 42
Antibiotic combinations
    and reduced toxicity, 167
    and renal sufficiency, 160
Antibiotic metabolism, drug effects on, 40
Antibiotic prophylactics in gastrointestinal surgery, 178
Antibiotic resistance, emergence during treatment, 5
Antibiotic toxicity, clinical manifestations of, 153
Antimicrobials and host defence mechanisms, 174

Bacteraemia, 3, 4
Bacterial cell envelope, 69
Bacterial endocarditis, length of treatment, 146
Bacteroides, 131
Biotransformation, 39

Calcium limitation, 84
Candida endocarditis, 143
Cell wall, gram-positive, 72
Cell wall, gram-negative, 73
Cephalosporins and aminoglycosides, 18
Chessboard titration, 57
Chloramphenicol, and penicillins, 25
Chloramphenicol inactivation, 100
Clostridium difficile, 6, 168
Clinical problems, 1
Clavulanic acid, 115
Clavulanic acid in treatment, 131
Cloxacillin and ampicillin, 110
Combined therapy, indications for, 4
Complementation, 55

Definitions of synergy, 10, 11
Distribution, interference with, 38
Drug metabolism, antibiotic effects on, 40
Dual activity, 56

Electrolyte disturbance, 155
Enterococci, 2
Enterocolitis, 166
Enzyme inhibitors, 99

Eradication of infection, 172
Excretion of antibiotics
  decrease of by other drugs, 41
  renal, 41
Experimental bacterial endocarditis, 141
Experimental bacterial meningitis, 139
Experimental models, 137

Fractional inhibitory concentration, 57
Folate metabolism, 87
Folate synthesis, 87
Fusidic acid, and penicillins, 20, 29

Gentamicin–carbenicillin interaction, 49

Haemophilus influenzae meningitis, 140
Hepatotoxicity, 155
Hydrophilic drugs, 74
Hydrophobic drugs, 75

Immunologically compromised patient, 7
Inoculum, size of, 14
Interaction, synergic, 6
Interactive chemotherapy, future uses of, 171
Intraperitoneal infection in mice, 138

Laboratory tests, interference by antibiotics, 47
β-Lactamase, 99, 104
  inhibition of, 55
    and bacterial synergy, 123
    by penicillins and cephalosporins, 108
    mechanism of, 119
  mammalian, 125
  occurrence of, 106
β-Lactamase inhibitors, 99, 105,
  miscellaneous, 113
  naturally occurring, 114
Life-threatening infection, 8
Listeria monocytogenes meningitis, 141
Lysis enhancement, 55

Mechanisms, of pharmacokinetic interactions, 36
Media constituents and antifolates, 91
Methodology, relevance of, 14
Minimum antibacterial concentration, 58
Mixed infections, 173

Nalidixic acid and rifampicin, 60
Nephrotoxicity, 154
  and antibiotic combinations, 161
Neurotoxicity, 155
Neutropenia, 7
Nutrient limitation, 78

"Penicillinase" inhibitors, 108
Penicillins
  and aminoglycosides, 18, 64
  and β-lactamase inhibitors, 19
  and chloramphenicol, 25
  and fusidic acid, 20, 29
Pharmacokinetic interactions, 35, 175
Pneumonia, with *Pseudomonas aeruginosa*, 5
Polymyxin and outer membrane, 77
Proteus mirabilis meningitis, 140
Pseudomembranous colitis, 6, 168
Pulmonary tuberculosis, 2
Purines, 90
Pyelonephritis, 7

Resistance,
  emergence of, 93, 97
  mutual suppression of, 56, 60
  prevention of, 173
Rifampicin and trimethoprim, 22, 27, 30

Shock, gram-negative, 6
Slime layer, 71
Staphylococcus aureus endocarditis, 142
Streptococcus faecalis endocarditis, 143
Streptococcus pneumoniae meningitis, 140
Streptococcus sanguis endocarditis, 142
Subacute bacterial endocarditis, 1, 9
Sub-MIC levels, 58
Sulphamethoxazole and trimethoprim, 29
Sulphonamides and trimethoprim, 21, 26
Synergism, clinical relevance of, 30
Synergistic activity, clinical needs for, 17
Synergistic combinations of antibiotics, clinical studies on, 17

Synergy,
  clinical relevance of, 13
  clinically obtainable, 15
  clinically useful, 15
  definitions of, 8, 10, 11
  laboratory methods, 53
  types of, 54

Thymineless mutants, 93
Toxicity,
    of antibiotic combinations, 151
  in animals, 158
    mechanisms of, 161
  prevention of, 173

Trimethoprim, 8
  and rifampicin, 22, 27, 30
  and sulphamethoxazole, 29, 59, 62
  and sulphonamides, 21, 26, 91
    mode of action of, 88
  resistance to, 96

Urinary bladder model, 59, 63, 64
Urinary tract infection, 8

Valve replacement, 10